Jane Marbel

D0436685

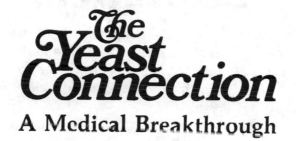

The Yeast Connection

A Medical Breakthrough

SECOND EDITION

By William G. Crook, M.D.

Illustrated by Cynthia P. Crook

Dedication

This book is gratefully and affectionately dedicated to my loyal secretary, Georgia Deaton, a skilled associate and perceptive collaborator. Thanks are due her not only for her contributions to this book, but for her help with numerous other endeavors during the past 27 years.

ISBN 0-933478-06-2

Library of Congress Catalog Number: 83-62508

Text © 1983, 1984 William G. Crook, M.D.
Illustrations © 1983, 1984 Cynthia P. Crook

All rights reserved. No part of this book may be reproduced or transmitted in any form or by any means, electronic or mechanical, including photocopying, storage and retrieval systems, without permission in writing from the publisher.

PROFESSIONAL BOOKS • P.O. Box 3494 • Jackson, Tennessee 38301

Acknowledgements

First, I thank C. Orian Truss, M.D. of Birmingham, Alabama. His brilliant pioneer observations on the *common yeast germ, Candida albicans,* alerted me to the possibility that candida could play an important role in causing health problems in many of my allergic patients . . . especially those with chemical sensitivity. I'm especially grateful to Dr. Truss for generously and patiently sharing his knowledge with me on countless occasions during the past three and one-half years.

Special thanks are also due to Sidney M. Baker, M.D., Head of the Gesell Institute of Human Development, New Haven, Connecticut. During the past four years, Dr. Baker's observations and concepts have greatly influenced me and my work with my patients, including those with yeast connected health problems. I'm grateful to many other physicians who have shared their knowledge and experiences with me, including especially Doctors Emanuel Cheraskin, Amos Christie, William Deamer, Larry Dickey, John Gerrard, Hobart Feldman, Alan Lieberman, John Maclennan, Marshall Mandell, Joseph McGovern, Joseph Miller, David Morris, James O'Shea, Robert Owen, Theron Randolph, Doris Rapp, William Rea, Douglas Sandberg, Frederic Speer, Del Stigler and Robert Stroud.

I'm also grateful to Doctor Elmer Cranton and to Betty Flora. Each of these individuals carefully reviewed my entire manuscript and made constructive suggestions for improving it. Thanks are also due to other helpful consultants, including Doctors Dor Brown, John Curlin, Harold Hedges, Phyllis Saifer, Morton Teich, Francis Waickman, Aubrey Worrell and Pat Connolly.

Special appreciation is due Rebecca Davis who helped significantly with the diet sections of this book, and to Susan and Sally Karlgaard, R.N. who served as invaluable consultants, coordinators and collaborators in completing the book.

I also appreciate the charming and delightful art work of my daughter, Cynthia, whose pictures make "The Yeast Connection" easy to understand.

I'm grateful, also, to other members of my staff, Ditzi Brittain, Brenda Harris, Nancy Moss, Bettye Patterson, Nell Sellers, Denny Spencer, Alice Spragins and Maggie Spragins who have helped me in numerous ways in putting this book together.

Finally, I appreciate the suggestions of many candida "victims" who have taught me a lot about yeast connected disease, including what helps them and what makes them worse. Included among these consultants are many of my own loyal patients as well as the patients of other physicians.

IMPORTANT NOTICE

This book describes relationships which have been observed between the common yeast germ *Candida albicans* and human illness. *I have written it to serve only as a general informational guide and reference source (for both professionals and non-professionals).* For obvious reasons I cannot assume the medical or legal responsibility of having the contents of this book considered as a prescription for anyone.

Treatment of illness, including those which appear to be yeast-connected must be supervised by a physician or other licensed health professional. Accordingly either you, or the professional who examines and treats you must take the responsibility for the uses made of this book.

William G. Crook, M.D.
September 7, 1983

Preface

to the First Edition

I finished medical school in 1942 and returned to my home town to practice in 1949. Beginning in 1955, I learned that a number of my patients improved when they stopped eating common foods, including milk, corn, wheat, egg and chocolate.

Soon afterward, pioneer allergist, Theron Randolph, taught me that many people with allergies and other chronic health problems suffered from the "chemical susceptibility" problem. And I learned that exposure to tobacco smoke, perfumes, colognes and petro-chemicals would cause troublesome (and at times disabling) symptoms in such patients.

Through the decade of the 60's and 70's, my interest grew in chronic illness caused by adverse reactions to foods and chemicals. So did my interest in nutrition, including vitamin and mineral deficiencies, and the adverse effects of sugar.

In the summer of 1979, I learned from C. Orian Truss of the relationship of the common yeast germ, *Candida albicans*, to many chronic illnesses. In the fall of 1979, I decided to try this approach on one of my difficult patients . . . a 41-year old woman (I'll call her Nancy Jones) with severe chronic hives, accompanied by mental confusion, fatigue and depression. I had struggled to help Nancy for over a year and nothing I did helped. Study and treatment at two university medical centers was similarly unsuccessful.

Six days after Nancy started on nystatin and a yeast-free, low-carbohydrate diet, her hives improved. Within a few weeks, her hives disappeared completely. She followed her diet and took nystatin for almost a year and her other symptoms also gradually improved. Recently, Nancy commented, "I'm perfectly well. I feel great . . . working every day. Nystatin and the diet helped tremendously. So did extra vitamins, especially vitamin B-12."

During the next six months, I treated an additional twenty patients using the special diet and nystatin. Nearly all were adults with complex health problems, including headache, fatigue, depression, recurrent vaginal infection, joint pain and sensitivity to chemical odors and additives. Almost without exception, they improved. And some improved dramatically.

During the past 3 years, my interest in Candida albicans and its relationship to human illness has grown rapidly. I've been able to help hundreds of my adult patients with symptoms ranging from headache to depression and from arthritis to multiple sclerosis using a candida control treatment program. Within the past year and a half, a number of my pediatric patients with chronic health problems, including hyperactive behavior and recurrent ear problems, have been helped by a similar program.

Yet, I've continued to be interested in factors other than yeasts which play a role in causing health problems in my patients. These include adverse reactions to specific foods, inhalants and chemicals, nutritional deficiencies and psychological factors.

But my recognition of "the yeast connection" has changed my life and my practice and has enabled me to help many, many patients conquer previously disabling illnesses.

This book is designed to make "The Yeast Connection" easily understood by individuals with chronic health problems. It is also directed toward physicians and other professionals who are interested or involved in treating patients with yeast-related illness.

Finally, I hope it will interest the public, including leaders in the field of business, labor, government and the media because I sincerely feel that recognition and appropriate management of yeast connected illness can play a major role in what I recently referred to as "The Coming Revolution in Medicine."[1]

This "revolution" will help physicians and their co-workers relieve much unnecessary suffering. It will also save patients, the government, business and industry (including the health insurance industry) billions of dollars.

Preface
to the Second Edition

As I worked to complete the manuscript of the first edition of *The Yeast Connection*, I consulted dozens of people who were knowledgeable and interested in human illness related to *Candida albicans. I also listened to my patients.*

Everyone I talked to agreed that diet and the unusually safe antifungal medication, nystatin, helped most people start on the road to recovery. But ideas differed as to exactly what the diet should consist of.

Experiences with nystatin, ketoconazole (Nizoral®), yogurt and other anti-candida treatment measures also were varied. Accordingly, when I finally "kissed my manuscript good-bye" and turned it over to my printer in September, 1983, I commented to a friend, "I have more questions than answers."

Trying to answer the question "What diet should I recommend?" challenged me and gave me many ambivalent feelings (see pages 67-69). For example, as I pointed out in the introduction to the section dealing with diet, I commented, *"Diets rich in complex car bohydrates (vegetables, whole grains and fruits) contribute to the good health of most people.* (pages 67-69).

Yet, C. Orian Truss, M.D., in discussing the dietary treatment of chronic candidiasis in his book, *The Missing Diagnosis*[52], said:

> "The first component of the 'avoidance' aspect of yeast control embodies certain modifications of the diet. Of the three classes of foods, yeasts ferment fat and protein poorly but thrive on carbohydrate. Limiting the intake of sweets and starches deprives the candida of the nutrient that allows its maximum multiplication.
>
> *"It's difficult to evaluate benefits from these dietary restrictions when other measures are simultaneously alleviating symptoms. But in theory as well as practice, diet is important, especially early in treatment. Occa-*

sional departures seem not to aggravate symptoms noticeably, in contrast to the continued high intake of these foods."

In conversations with me on several occasions, Dr. Truss confirmed these observations and in most of his patients he recommends a diet which contains only 60 to 80 grams of carbohydrate each day. Then, after 2 to 4 months, as his patients improve, he suggests that carbohydrates be cautiously increased.

In November, 1983, I sent a questionnaire to a number of practicing physicians who are treating patients with yeast-connected illness.† Most recommended that carbohydrates, initially, be restricted to 60 to 100 grams. *However, all of these physicians felt that diets must be individualized to suit the unique needs of each patient.*

One knowledgeable physician with a background in nutrition and biochemistry commented, "Avoiding sugars, corn syrup, white flour products and other refined and processed carbohydrates is essential. Yet I do not recommend avoiding the good complex carbohydrates found in whole grains and fruits unless a person doesn't tolerate them."

In December, 1983, I interviewed John W. Rippon, Ph.D., of the University of Chicago, an authority on yeasts and molds. In discussing diets to discourage the multiplication of yeasts, Dr. Rippon commented,

> "Yeasts thrive on the simple carbohydrates including sugar, syrup and honey. Fruits also encourage yeast growth. Vegetables (even those high in carbohydrates) and whole grains do not. However, more research should be done to further confirm these observations."

I was so impressed with Dr. Rippon's knowledge and expertise I felt I should include his viewpoint in this second edition of *The Yeast Connection.* Because of what I learned from him and from others (including my patients), I made significant changes in my diet recommendations. I continued to emphasize the importance of avoiding sugars and foods containing yeasts and molds. *I also advised that fruits and milk be avoided during the early weeks of treatment* (see pages 42-43, 75, 89, 95-110, 117-120 and 298-300).

I revised and updated my comments on the pre-menstrual syndrome (page 187) and included comments by two practicing gynecologists who have found that an anti-candida treatment program has helped many of their PMS patients. I included a report by Dr.

Alan Levin of San Francisco describing the dramatic response of a child with autism to anti-candida therapy using high doses of Nizoral® .

In section E, Chapter 36, *Other Helpful Information,* under the heading *Mobilizing Your Health Resources,* I emphasized the importance of finding a knowledgeable and caring physician as well as utilizing faith, hope and prayer. In this chapter I also listed and briefly described 35 sources of information, help and support for those with yeast-connected health disorders and those with illnesses related to nutritional, allergic or environmental causes.

In Chapter 37, *What You Can Do If Your Physician Is Unaware of The Yeast Connection,* I made a number of suggestions which I hope you'll find useful (including directions for making yogurt). In this chapter I also discussed the rapidly burgeoning consumer interest in *alternative* or *complementary medicine* in North America and Great Britain. And I briefly reviewed comments on this subject from *The New England Journal of Medicine,* the *London Times,* Marilyn Ferguson and John Naisbitt.

I put together a chapter entitled "Potpourri" (Chapter 39). In this chapter are new materials including: A summary of clinical observations of twelve practicing physicians who are using anti-candida therapy; new methods of studying and treating patients with mold sensitivity; notes on laboratory studies that may help; comments on candida toxins; selenium and other anti-oxidants. I also discussed garlic, milk and exercise.

I added additional material on autism, urticaria, the premenstrual syndrome (PMS), and commented on the role of candida in marital problems and divorce. I discussed the possible toxicity of aspartame and mercury/amalgam dental fillings.

I also defined and commented on orthomolecular medicine and added suggestions on readily available sources of information on nutrition. Finally, I added a much needed twenty-two page Index.

Everyone interested in yeast-connected illness agrees that more research is needed. So in my postscript I added a special plea to "anyone and everyone" to lend financial support to the Critical Illness Research Foundation (see page 302)

Are Your Health Problems Yeast-Connected?

	YES	NO
1. Have you taken repeated "rounds" of antibiotic drugs?	☐	☐
2. Have you been troubled by premenstrual tension, abdominal pain, menstrual problems, vaginitis, prostatitis, or loss of sexual interest?	☐	☐
3. Does exposure to tobacco, perfume and other chemical odors provoke moderate to severe symptoms?	☐	☐
4. Do you crave sugar, breads or alcoholic beverages?	☐	☐
5. Are you bothered by recurrent digestive symptoms?	☐	☐
6. Are you bothered by fatigue, depression, poor memory, or "nerves"?	☐	☐
7. Are you bothered by hives, psoriasis, or other chronic skin rashes?	☐	☐
8. Have you ever taken birth control pills?	☐	☐
9. Are you bothered by headaches, muscle and joint pains or incoordination?	☐	☐
10. Do you feel bad all over, yet the cause hasn't been found?	☐	☐

If you have 3 or 4 "yes" answers, yeasts *possibly* play a role in causing your symptoms.

If you have 5, 6, or 7 "yes" answers, yeast *probably* play a role in causing your symptoms.

If you have 8, 9 or 10 "yes" answers, your symptoms are *almost certainly* yeast-connected.

Copyright ©1983, William G. Crook, M.D.

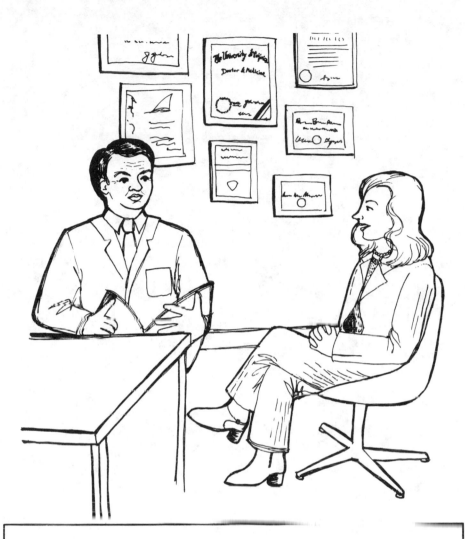

Before assuming your symptoms are caused or triggered by the common yeast germ, *Candida albicans*, go to your physician for a careful history and physical examination and appropriate laboratory studies or tests. An examination is important because many other disorders can cause similar symptoms.

However, if a careful check-up doesn't reveal the cause for your symptoms, and your medical history (as described in this book) is "typical," it's possible or even probable that your health problems are yeast connected.

What This Book Is All About

If you (or your child) are bothered by . . .

- Extreme fatigue or lethargy (the feeling of being drained)
- Depression
- Inability to concentrate
- Headaches
- Skin problems (such as hives, athlete's foot, fungous infection of the nails, jock itch, psoriasis or other chronic skin rashes)
- Gastrointestinal symptoms (especially constipation, abdominal pain, diarrhea, gas or bloating)
- Symptoms involving your reproductive organs
- Muscular and nervous system symptoms (including aching or swelling in your muscles and joints, numbness, burning or tingling, muscle weakness or paralysis)
- Respiratory symptoms
- Hyperactivity and recurrent ear problems . . .

go to your doctor for a careful checkup, including a history and physical examination, complete blood count, urinalysis, and tuberculin test. Depending on the nature and duration of your complaints and the findings on your initial examination, your physician may feel that other tests and studies are necessary.

Yeast-connected health problems occur in people of all ages and both sexes. However, women are more apt to be affected. Yeasts are especially apt to play a role in causing your health problems if you:

1. Feel bad "all over," yet the cause can't be identified and treatment of many kinds hasn't helped.
2. Have taken prolonged courses of broad-spectrum antibiotic drugs, including the tetracyclines (Sumycin® Panmycin®, Vibramycin®, Minocin®, etc), ampicillin, amoxicillin, the

cephalosporins (Keflex®, Ceclor®, etc.), and sulfonamide drugs, including Septra® and Bactrim®.

3. Have consumed diets containing a lot of yeast and sugar.
4. Crave sweets.
5. Crave other carbohydrates, especially breads and pizza.
6. Notice that sweets make your symptoms worse or give you a "pick-up," followed by a "let-down."
7. Have symptoms which make you feel you're bothered by "hypoglycemia," yet tests may fail to confirm such a diagnosis.
8. Crave alcohol.
9. Have taken birth control pills, prednisone, Decadron® or other corticosteroid drugs.
10. Have had multiple pregnancies.
11. Have been troubled by recurrent problems related to your reproductive organs, including abdominal pain, vaginal infection or discomfort, premenstrual tension, menstrual irregularities, prostatitis or impotence.
12. Are bothered by persistent or recurrent symptoms involving your digestive and nervous systems.
13. Have been bothered by persistent or recurrent athlete's foot, fungous infection of the nails or "jock itch."
14. Feel bad on damp days or in moldy places.
15. Are made ill when exposed to perfumes, tobacco smoke and other chemicals.

This book is written for patients, professionals and para-professionals, and for the public at large. **Section A** explains why yeast-connected illness develops and how it can be suspected and identified. This section also deals with treatment, and a question and answer format discusses the use of nystatin and other anti-fungal medication.

Diet plays a major role in the successful management of yeast-connected illness. Accordingly, **Section B** includes a detailed discussion of the foods which should be eaten and those which must be avoided. Illustrations and menus are provided to make dietary instructions easier to follow.

Section C emphasizes that "unwellness" or ill health is rarely (if ever) due only to yeasts (or to any other single cause). Instead, illness develops because of a web of interacting causes. Accordingly, individuals with yeast-connected illness (and the professionals and para-professionals who work with them) must pay attention to the many other factors which determine whether a person is sick or well. Simple illustrations are again used to clarify concepts and instructions.

Section D discusses the many and varied manifestations of yeast-connected illness. Featured in this section is an extensive discussion of yeast-connected illness in women, men, young children and teen-agers. Also featured is a discussion of the relationship of yeasts to a number of baffling and supposedly incurable diseases, including multiple sclerosis, schizophrenia, arthritis, psoriasis and systemic lupus erythematosus. Illustrative patient histories are presented and are an important part of this section.

In **Section E**, you'll find a varied group of comments and suggestions that may help you overcome your yeast-connected health problems. Many items listed are "routine" instructions and their listing in this section serves as a reminder or check list. Others are based on suggestions I've obtained from many sources, including my patients and other professionals. I also briefly summarize the discussions of the *Informal Conference on Candida Albicans and Its Relationship to Human Illness* held in Dallas, Texas in July, 1982.

The Yeast Connection . . . A Vicious Cycle

Antibiotics, especially broad spectrum antibiotics, kill "friendly germs" while they're killing enemies. And when friendly germs are knocked out, yeast germs (*Candida albicans*) multiply.

Diets rich in carbohydrates and yeasts, birth control pills, cortisone and other drugs also stimulate yeast growth.

Large numbers of yeasts weaken your immune system. Your immune system is also affected adversely by nutritional deficiencies and sugar consumption, and by exposure to environmental molds and chemicals (such as formaldehyde, petrochemicals, perfume and tobacco.)

When your immune system is compromised and your resistance is lessened, you may feel bad "all over" and develop respiratory, digestive and other symptoms. And you're apt to develop adverse reactions to additional foods, inhalants and chemicals. As a part of these reactions, mucous membranes throughout your body swell and you develop infections caused by bacteria and viruses that a strong immune system would ordinarily conquer.

When you develop an infection, you're apt to be given "broad spectrum" antibiotics. Such antibiotics, while at times essential, promote the growth of *Candida albicans* which depresses your immune system. And your health problems continue until the vicious cycle is interupted by a comprehensive treatment program designed to decrease the growth of *Candida albicans* and increase your resistance.

THE YEAST CONNECTION...A VICIOUS CYCLE

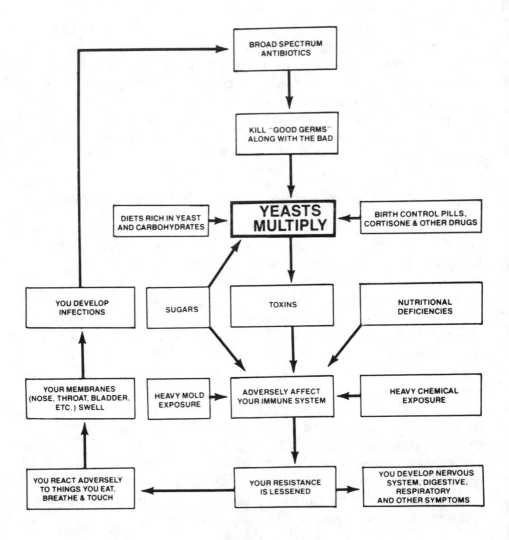

Table Of Contents

SECTION A:
How You Suspect, Identify and Treat Yeast-Connected Illness

1 What Are Yeasts?.. 3
2 A Typical Patient, Janet, Tells Her Story................. 5
3 About Your Immune System and How Yeasts
Make You Sick.........,,,,,............................ 9

• How a Strong Immune System Protects You • Yeast Germs Normally Live in Your Body • When Yeasts Multiply, They Weaken Your Immune System • When Your Immune System Loses Strength, You Develop Health Problems • Yeasts Are Only One of the Factors Which Weaken Your Immune System • Many Different Things Encourage Yeast Growth

4 You Can Suspect That Candida Plays a Role in
Making You Sick, IF.................................... 17
5 Identifying The Candida Problem 27
6 Candida Questionnaire and Score Sheet 29
7 Treating Your Candida Problem 35
8 Overcoming Yeast-connected Illness .
  Questions and Answers............................... 39
9 More About Yeasts, Molds and Other Fungi 55

• Sources of Mold in Homes • Controlling Yeasts and Molds: Avoid Molds at Home and at Work; Avoid Antibiotics; Avoid "The Pill"; Treat Your Home with Formaldehyde Vapors?

SECTION B:
To Control Candida, You Must Change Your Diet

10 Introduction 57
11 The Candida Control Diet............................. 75

• Foods You Can Eat • Foods You Must Avoid • Meal Suggestions • Shopping Tips • Food Sources • Additional Helpful Suggestions

12 The Low Carbohydrate Diet 95
   • Foods You Can Eat Freely • Foods You Can Eat Cautiously • Meal
   Suggestions • Low Carbohydrate 7-Day Meal Plan
13 Yeast Free Recipes 111
14 Fruit-Free, Sugar-Free, Yeast-Free, Diet 117
   •The Yeast-Free, Fruit-Free, Sugar-Free, Grain-Free, Nut-Free, Milk-
   Free Diet
15 Ideas for Breakfast and Eating on the Run 121
16 If Sugar is a No-No, What Can I Use? 123
17 Food Allergies 127

SECTION C:
Keeping Candida Under Control
Requires More Than Medication and a Special Diet

18 Introduction 133
19 To Overcome Candida and Enjoy Good Physical,
   Mental and Emotional Health: 137
   • You Must Seek These Vital Nutrients • You Must Avoid . . .
   • You Must Be Treated for Allergies and Infections • You Need a
   Favorable Environment
20 The Causes of Illness Resemble a Web 145
21 Is Your Camel's Load Too Heavy? 147
22 The Puzzle of Chronic Illness 149
23 Chemicals May Play a Role in Making You Sick 151
24 How Chemicals Make You Sick 157
25 When Candida is Treated, Your Chemical
   Sensitivity Will Often Improve 159
26 About Your Immune System and How It
   Protects You 163
27 Labeling Diseases Isn't the Way We Should Go 167
28 Every Part of Your Body is Connected
   to Every Other Part 173

SECTION D:
Manifestations of Yeast-Connected Illness

29 Health Problems of Women 179
   • A Special Word About PMS (Premenstrual Syndrome) • Why
   Yeast-Connected Illness Occurs More in Women, Especially Young
   Women
30 Men, Too, Develop Yeast-Connected Health Problems 191

31 Health Problems of Children 195
   •Ear Problems of Children . . . Isn't There a Better Answer?
32 Physical and Mental Problems of Teenagers 213
33 Does Candida Cause Multiple Sclerosis, Psoriasis,
   Arthritis or Schizophrenia? 219
34 Can Candida Albicans Make a Tee-Totaler Drunk? 229
35 Overcoming Yeast-connected Illness Isn't Always Easy 231

SECTION E:
Other Helpful Information

36 Miscellaneous Measures That May Help You 243

   • Low Carbohydrate Diet • Hidden Food Allergies • Rotated Diets
   • Multivitamin and Mineral Supplements • Vitamin C • Cal-
   cium/Magnesium Supplements • Essential Fatty Acids • Iron Sup-
   plements • Intravaginal Nystatin • Sniffing or Inhaling Nystatin •
   Nystatin enemas • Die-Off Reactions Following Nystatin • Mold
   Control In Your Home • Lessen Your Exposure To Chemicals • Try
   The Herbal Remedy Taheebo Tea • Yogurt • Hormone Imbalance •
   Treat The Marital Partner and/or Other Family Members • Immu-
   notherapy • Air Ionizers • Certain Foods Kill or Inhibit Candida •
   Fruit and Grain-Induced Reactions • Large Doses of Vitamin A •
   Wood Burning Stoves and Fireplaces May Aggravate Yeast-
   Connected Symptoms • Digestive Enzymes • Clotrimazole • Clean-
   ing Foods • Mobilizing Your Health Resources • Other Sources of
   Information

37. What You Can Do If Your Physician Is Unaware
   Of The Yeast Connection 265
38 Summary of the 1982 Dallas Informal Conference 271
39 Potpourri 277

   • Observations of Practicing Physicians • Amphotericin B: A
   Special Report to Physicians • Other Candida Species May Cause
   Problems • New Methods of Studying and Treating Patients with
   Mold Sensitivity • Selenium and Other Antioxidants • Laboratory
   Studies May Help • Yeast Toxins • Yeast-connected Urticaria
   • More on Candida and Autism (An Anecdotal Report) • More on
   PMS • Marital Problems and Divorce • Garlic May Help Control
   Yeasts • More on Amino Acids • Comments on Milk • Exercise
   • More on Aspartame • Mercury/Amalgam Toxicity • What Does
   "Orthomolecular" Mean? • More on Nutrition

40 Postscript 301
41 References 303
42 Reading List 309
General Index 315

"Sit down before a fact, as a little child, be prepared to give up every preconceived notion, follow humbly wherever and to whatever abyss nature leads or you shall learn nothing."

Thomas Huxley

"It is very unscientific not to have an open mind."

E. William Rosenberg, M.D.

Section A

How you suspect,
identify and treat
yeast-connected
illness.

What are yeasts?

Yeasts are single cell fungi which belong to the vegetable kingdom. And like their "cousins" the molds, they live all around you. And one family of yeasts, "Candida albicans", normally lives in your body and more especially in your intestines and other parts of your digestive tract.

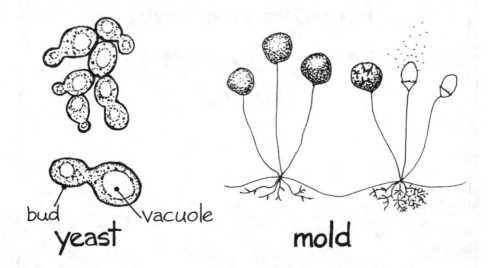

bud vacuole
yeast   **mold**

What Are Yeasts?

In his book, *Medical Mycology*,[2] John Willard Rippon, Ph.D. said in effect:

> "Yeasts (including *Candida albicans*) are mild mannered creatures incapable of producing infection in the normal healthy individual. They only cause trouble in the person with weakened defenses.
> . . . "The severity of the disease will depend on how weak a person's resistance is, rather than on any disease-producing properties exhibited by the fungus . . . . Because of its rapid ability to make itself at home on mucous membranes (the medical term is "colonize") and take advantage of many types of host alterations, the clinical manifestations of candida infection are exceedingly variable . . . . *Candida albicans accounts for the vast majority of diseases caused by the yeast.*"

In his continuing discussion, Dr. Rippon tells about the different types and classifications of the various yeasts, including common brewer's and baker's yeasts, as well as the yeasts found in beer, ale and wine. Still other yeasts are lactose fermenters and are associated with the preparation of fermented milk beverages.

Hippocrates described one type of yeast infection, *thrush*, in debilitated patients and the presence of this clinical condition has been recognized for centuries. Galen described it as a common occurrence in children, particularly sickly children. Textbooks of pediatrics in the 1700's also described thrush and in the 1800's it was first noted to be acquired through passage of the baby through the mother's womb.

A confusing number of different names have been applied to this same yeast organism we know as *Candida albicans*. These have included '*Oidium albicans*', '*Saccaromyces albicans*' and '*Monilia albicans*'. Apparently different observers in different countries developed their own pet names.

According to Rippon, vaginal yeast infection (candidiasis) was first described by Wilkinson in 1849. Systemic disease caused by candida was described in a debilitated patient in 1861 and on a number of occasions thereafter during the 19th century.

Candida infections of the nails were first described in 1904, skin disease in 1907, and candida cystitis in 1910. Chronic mucocutaneous disease was probably first described in 1909. By the early 1940's, it thus became evident that candidiasis was the most variable of the fungous infections. Statistically it was a common infecting agent of the skin, mucosa and vagina; yet it was rarely found to cause serious systemic disease.

In his continuing discussion, Rippon commented,

> "A revival of interest in systemic candidiasis took place after 1940. The occurrence of candidiasis as a sequel to the use of antibacterial antibiotics, particularly broad spectrum antibiotics, evoked a great surge of research . . . Presently, candida is recognized as one of the most frequently encountered fungal opportunists and is now regarded as the commonest cause of serious fungal disease."

Another recent informative book, *Candida and Candidosis*,[3] by British microbiologist, F.C. Odds, comprehensively covers *Candida albicans* and other candida species. According to Dr. Odds, 200 to 300 scientific articles on candida appear annually and his book lists 2,265 references. Serious students of yeast-connected illness will find this book to be a treasure house of information.

Yet, in spite of these thousands of scientific articles on Candida albicans, until the first paper by C. Orian Truss[†], there were only occasional references in the medical literature[††] suggesting that usually harmless yeast organisms could be related to so many different medical disorders.

---

† Presented at the Eighth Annual Scientific Symposium of the Academy of Orthomolecular Psychiatry held in Toronto, April 30 - May 1, 1977, and published in the *Journal of Orthomolecular Psychiatry*, 7:17-37, 1978 (Publications office: 2231 Broad Street, Saskatchewan, Canada). Two subsequent papers in the same journal extended and clarified Truss' brilliant pioneer observations and concepts. All three of these papers are reprinted in the book, THE MISSING DIAGNOSIS, published by Truss in January, 1983. (Information about ordering this book can be obtained by writing to: THE MISSING DIAGNOSIS, P.O. Box 26508, Birmingham, Alabama 35226.)

†† In November, 1983, Drs. Lawrence Dickey and Francis Waickman pointed out that Alfred V. Zamm, M.D. of Kingston, New York, had published original observations on the role of Candida albicans in chronic urticaria and other allergies and diseases of obscure cause. Dr. Zamm's recommended program of management included a yeast free diet and a therapeutic trial of nystatin. His observations were presented in part at the annual meeting of the Society for Clinical Ecology in Chicago December 12, 1970, and were subsequently published in a series of articles in CUTIS (January and February, 1972 and May, 1973) and in the book CLINICAL ECOLOGY (see Reading List page 309).

A Typical Patient, Janet, Tells Her Story

During the past 4 years, I've seen hundreds of patients (especially young women) with yeast-connected health problems. Here's a typical story as recorded by 33-year-old Janet:†

"I'm ready to find out if it's 'all in my head' and my symptoms are due to 'just getting older' or whether there's something that's really making me feel sick.

"All my childhood, I suffered with stomach problems which were usually blamed on 'nerves.' But when my children developed allergies, I began to suspect that allergies were part of my trouble, too.

"After my first child was born (1976), I was troubled by painful aches in my fingers and knees for 2 or 3 months. When my mother suggested I quit dipping the baby's diapers and quit using Clorox®, the aches went away.

"About a year later, I developed a strange swelling in my ankles and feet which caused enough pain to prevent walking. I couldn't even get my shoes on. So I went to an orthopedic surgeon (my dad, a physician, was out of the country). Although he found no reason for the swelling, he did give me medicine. Gradually the swelling subsided.

"I began having headaches, dizziness, nausea, sore throat and earaches in the fall of 1980. My doctor put me on several antihistamines and intermittent antibiotics. But because I hate to depend on medicine, in the fall of 1981, I decided to eliminate coffee, tea, milk, orange juice, colas and chocolate because of food-induced reactions I'd seen in my children.

"Food elimination helped to some degree, but during the winter and spring I was troubled by persistent night cough and a tickle in my throat. I took another round of antibiotics which helped temporarily, but then my symptoms returned.

"Last summer, after a short exposure to paint, I felt sick with generalized aching, symptoms of a cold and hurting in my chest. From time to time, I would develop what seemed like the flu but it would only last one day. As I tried to figure it out, I remembered that I had used Clorox® and Comet®.

---

† This patient was reported in my recent article in the *Journal of the Tennessee State Medical Association.*[1]

"On the last two occasions when I've had my teeth filled, the reaction I experienced scared me and my dentist, too. Injections of Lidocaine® to deaden my gum made me tingle and feel light-headed, confused and fatigued. Codein also caused adverse effects.

"This spring, I've developed bladder problems; two infections and frequent urination. I've also been unable to empty my bladder without hard pushing. These symptoms took me to a urologist who diagnosed it as 'a small urethra and spasm'. He dilated me and gave me medicine. Incidentally, frequent urination had been a part of my life, but not the pressure. (I have even wet the bed since I've been married.)

"I also am bothered by nervousness, fatigue, puffiness of my fingers, bloating, excessive weight gain and breast soreness during the week before my period."

When I first saw Janet on July 10, 1982, she looked tired and dark circles under her eyes accentuated the appearance of fatigue. Her nasal membranes appeared swollen and lavender in color, and a transverse crease extended acrooss her nose. A review of her diet showed that while she ate some "good foods," she "loved sweets," including sugar-sweetened cereals, ice cream, Mountain Dew® and Oreo® cookies.

A further review of Janet's history revealed that she had taken antibiotics on five occasions during the last year. Moreover, she had been treated for vaginal yeast infection on four occasions in less than 12 months. Other symptoms included swelling, weight gain, breast soreness, loss of sexual feeling and increased fatigue during the week before the beginning of her menstrual period.

Because of Janet's respiratory symptoms, I carried out limited allergy testing to the common inhalants. Much to my surprise, there were no significant reactions. So because her history strongly suggested yeast-related illness, I prescribed nystatin, 1-million units (¼ teaspoon of powder) four times a day, and a yeast free, low carbohydrate diet. Two weeks after beginning treatment, Janet reported:

"I'm much better. My ears are better, my night cough and bladder symptoms are gone. My energy level has improved significantly and I no longer feel bloated."

Nystatin and dietary treatment were continued, and a yeast-free vitamin/mineral preparation was added along with supplemental essential fatty acids, calcium lactate and magnesium oxide.

In the ensuing months, Janet steadily improved. However, she would notice a flareup of her symptoms whenever she ate foods containing sugar or yeast, or when she was exposed to chemicals. She also found that a dose of ½ teaspoon of nystatin, 4 times a day, was needed for maximal symptom relief; when she cut the dose in half, her generalized aching returned.

At a follow-up visit on March 8, 1983, eight months after starting on her treatment program, Janet reported:

> "I've had an excellent winter. I'm symptom-free and well, except when I cheat on my diet."

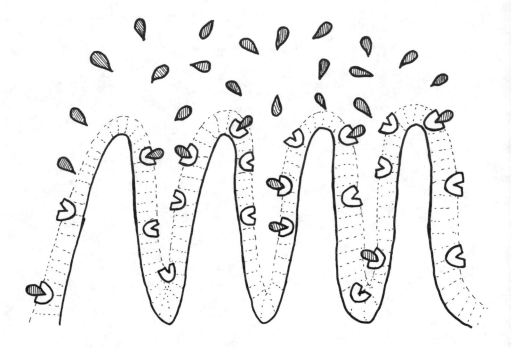

🌢 Attacker

♡ Defender

⬤ Immune Complex

3

About Your Immune System And How Yeasts Make You Sick

How A Strong Immune System Protects You

Your immune system protects you by automatically recognizing all sorts of enemies. Using many marvelous methods, it neutralizes, conquers or eliminates these enemies.

Your immune system is composed of many defenders including "antibodies" and different kinds of white blood cells. These protective substances might be compared to the United States Army, Navy, Marines or Air Force.

Fortifications or mechanical barriers (including your skin and mucous membranes) help keep invaders out. These mucous membranes ("MM's") line the interior cavities and passageways of your body, including your digestive tract, your respiratory tract, your genito-urinary tract and your eyes. Just below their surface are mucous-secreting glands which work like plastic "squeeze bottles."

These glands help protect your delicate membranes by coating them with mucus. And when dust, dirt, bacterial, viruses, chemicals or other substances try to invade or penetrate, the mucus provides a mechanical barrier.

Your MM's are also coated or "painted" with many different *antibodies,* including "secretory IgA" (a special type of gamma globulin or *immunoglobulin* . . . one of your immune system's important soldiers). When your lining membranes become inflamed, other *immunoglobulins,* including IgG, are found in the secretion.

The surface area of the intestinal membrane is as large as a tennis court. But rather than being a flat, smooth surface, it looks like the

9

coast of Norway. When yeast germs, toxins or other enemies (antigens) try to break through your MM's, your defenders (antibodies) combine with them. The resulting antigen/antibody complexes on the surface of your MM's are know as *immune complexes*.

Yeast Germs Normally Live In Your Body

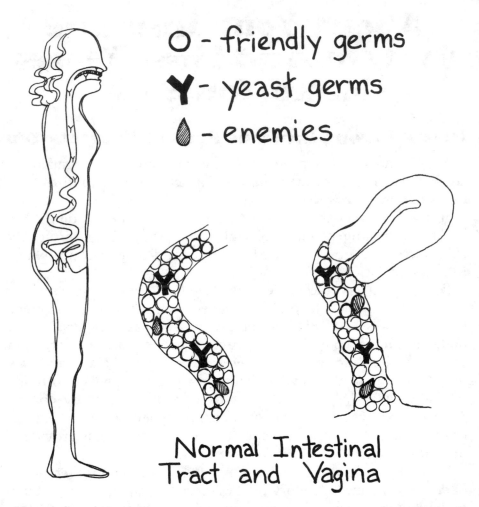

O – friendly germs
Y – yeast germs
⬤ – enemies

Normal Intestinal Tract and Vagina

A few families of yeast germs normally live on your mucous membranes, along with billions of friendly germs. (Yeasts especially feel at home in the warm, dark recesses of your digestive tract and your vagina.) Unfriendly bacteria, viruses, allergens and other enemies also find their way into these and other membrane-lined passage-ways and cavities, including your respiratory tract. But when your immune system is strong, they aren't able to get through into your deeper tissues or blood stream and make you sick.

When Yeasts Multiply
They Weaken Your Immune System

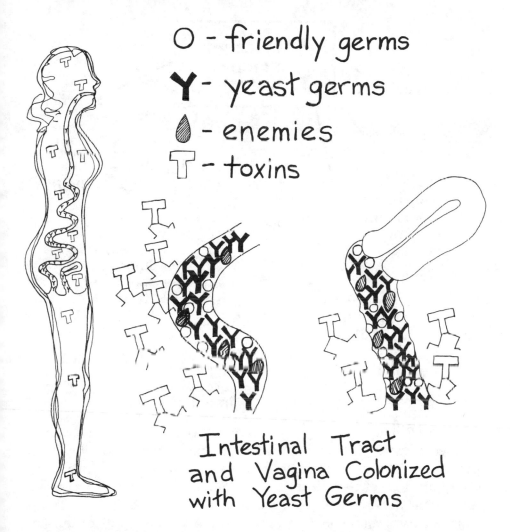

O – friendly germs

Y – yeast germs

◊ – enemies

T – toxins

Intestinal Tract and Vagina Colonized with Yeast Germs

When you take antibiotics, especially if you take them repeatedly, many of the friendly germs in your body (especially those in your digestive tract) are "wiped out." Since yeasts aren't harmed by these antibiotics, they spread out and raise large families (the medical term is "colonization").

When yeasts multiply, they put out toxins which circulate through your body, weaken your defenders and make you sick.

When Your Immune System Loses Strength, You Develop Health Problems

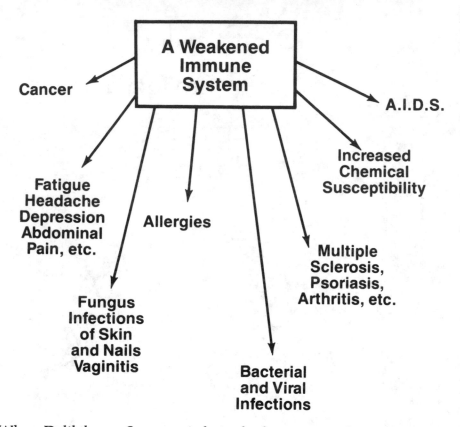

When Delilah cut Sampson's hair, he became weak. In a similar manner, yeast toxins weaken your immune system; and when your immune system loses strength, you develop many health problems. You're apt to feel bad all over and complain of fatigue, headache, depression, nervousness, abdominal pain and other digestive symptoms. And you may develop yeast or fungous infections of the skin and nails, or of moist areas or cavities of your body, including especially your vagina. You may be bothered by allergies of various sorts and become more susceptible to bacterial and viral infections.

You may also be troubled by arthritis, multiple sclerosis, psoriasis or other serious disorders and show an increased susceptibility to environmental chemicals.

When a person's immune system isn't functioning properly, other even more serious disorders may develop, including cancer† and the acquired immune deficiency syndrome . . ."AIDS".†

Yeasts Are Only One Of The Factors Which Weaken Your Immune System

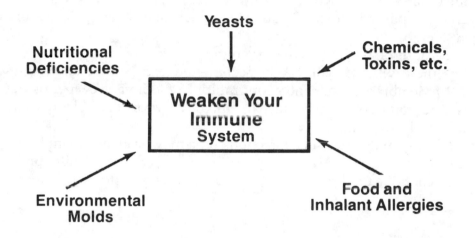

YEAST OVERGROWTH WEAKENS YOUR IMMUNE SYSTEM. Yet, it is only one of many factors. *Nutritional deficiencies* caused by inadequate intake and/or poor absorption of essential amino acids, essential fatty acids, complex carbohydrates, vitamins and minerals also weaken your immune system.

So do *environmental chemicals.* Included among these are home, industrial and farm chemicals and poisons, tobacco, lead, cadmium, mercury and many others.

Food and inhalant allergies, or a heavy load of *environmental molds,* also adversely affect your immune system.

---

†Could either of these disorders be yeast-connected? I do not know. Yet it is logical to assume that they could be because they occur in persons with weakened immune systems. Moreover, Truss recently commented, "Candida albicans seems to be at least one agent capable of at least a depressing, and perhaps a destructive effect on the immune system. Until the cause of the AIDS problem is uncovered, any approach would seem to be worth considering in a situation of such urgency." (Truss, C.O.: (Letters) *Journal of Orthomolecular Psychiatry*, Vol. 12, #1, 1983, p. 37.)

Many Different Things Encourage Yeast Growth.

Twentieth century diets (1) which are rich in sugar and yeast, birth control pills (2) and pregnancy (3) encourage yeast growth. So do hormonal changes (4) during each menstrual cycle. But antibiotic drugs (5), especially "broad spectrum" antibiotics, make yeasts grow like grass and weeds after a summer rainy spell. Such drugs destroy good germs while they're killing bad ones. Yeasts then multiply.

Although yeasts (6) are found normally in your body, when your immune system is strong they don't bother you. But when they increase in number, toxins (7) are released which weaken your immune system (8).

Because of your weakened immune system, the defenders which line the cavities of your body become ineffective. (See, also pages 8-9.) Membranes swell and germs multiply and invade deeper tissues (9). So you develop nose, throat, sinus, ear, bronchial, bladder and other infections (10).

When you develop such infections, you may be given an antibiotic (5) which promotes additional yeast growth (6). So your health problems continue until the cycle is interrupted by appropriate treatment.

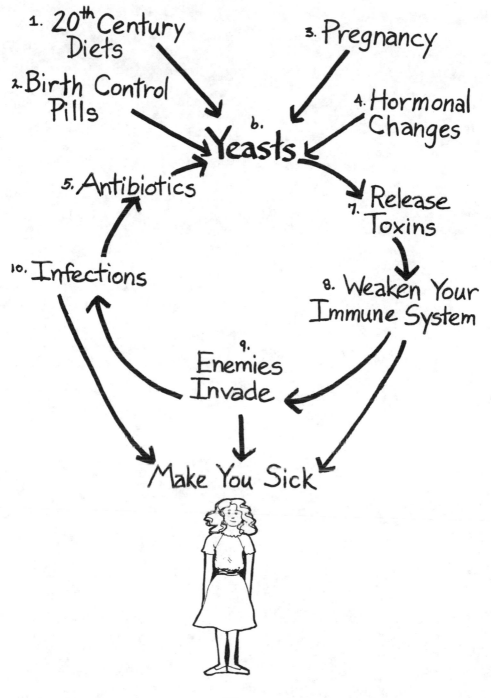

1. 20ᵗʰ Century Diets
2. Birth Control Pills
3. Pregnancy
4. Hormonal Changes
5. Antibiotics
6. Yeasts
7. Release Toxins
8. Weaken Your Immune System
9. Enemies Invade
10. Infections

Make You Sick

You Can Suspect That Candida Plays A Role In Making You Sick If . . .

you've taken antibiotics for acne

Prescription

R Tetracycline 250 mg.
#300

Sig: Take 1 capsule twice daily for 6 months.

Fred Nore, MD

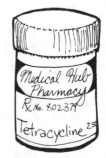

Medical Hub Pharmacy
R No. 802379
Tetracycline 250

**or prolonged or repeated
courses of
antibiotics**

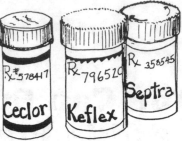

for 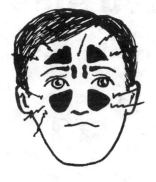 **sinusitis**

bronchitis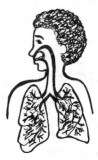

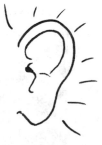 **urinary
or ear infections**

you've taken birth control pills†

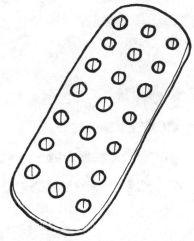

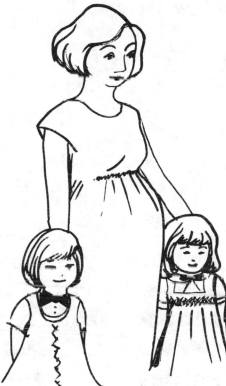

or have been pregnant†

---

†Birth control pills and pregnancy stimulate growth of the yeast germ.

you've taken cortisone, prednisone or other corticosteroids

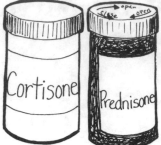

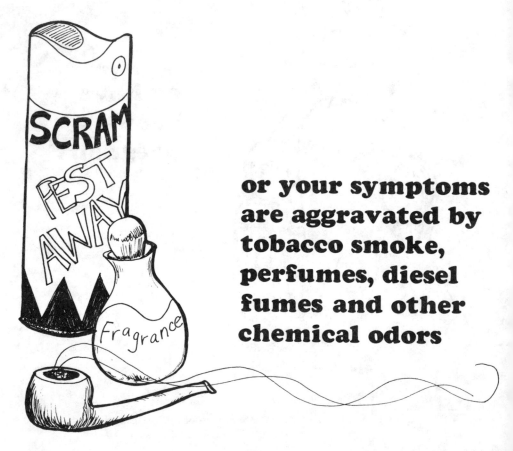

or your symptoms are aggravated by tobacco smoke, perfumes, diesel fumes and other chemical odors

you feel tired, lethargic, drained or depressed

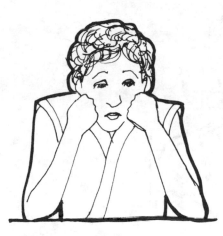

you're bothered by all sorts of other nervous system symptoms, including poor memory, feelings of unreality, irritability, headache or inability to concentrate

When *is* my next appointment ???

or . . .

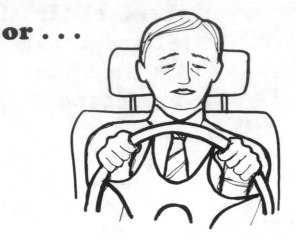

inappropriate drowsiness

numbness, tingling and muscle weakness

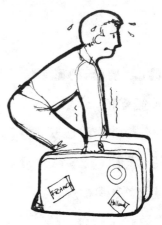

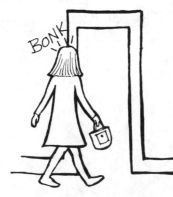

incoordination

you've been troubled by recurrent vaginal yeast infections or other disorders involving the sex organs or urinary system

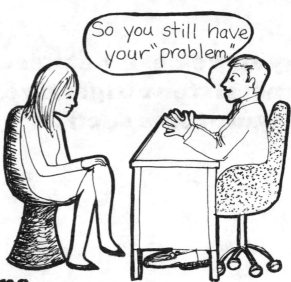

So you still have your "problem."

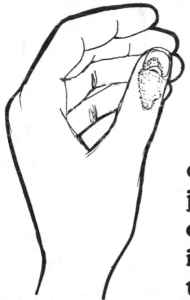

or athlete's foot, jock itch and other fungous infections of the skin

you've been bothered by
persistent digestive
symptoms such as

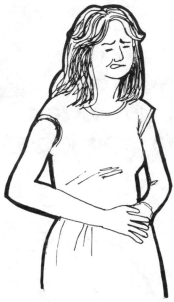

heartburn,
indigestion,
bloating,
abdominal pain,
gas,
constipation,
diarrhea,

you're bothered by other
troublesome symptoms such as
pain or swelling
of your joints,
nasal congestion,
recurrent sore
throats, cough,

pain or tightness
in your chest,
spots in front
of your eyes,
or blurred
vision, fluid
in your ears
or just
feeling "lousy"

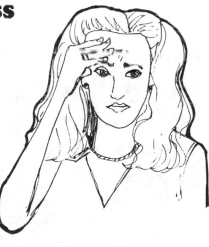

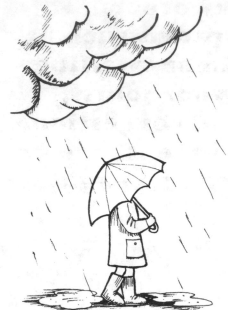

your symptoms flare up on damp days or in moldy places

or when you eat or drink foods which promote yeast growth

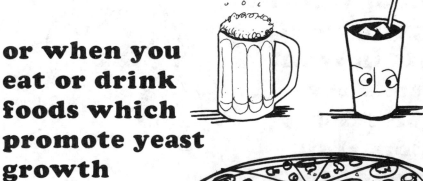

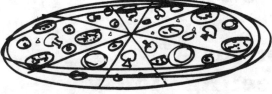

5

Identifying The Candida Problem

**Do tests help?
No . . .
or not much.**

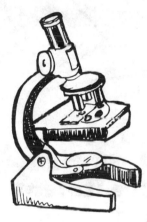

**Here's why: Candida germs
live in every person's body . . .
especially on the mucous
membranes. Accordingly
vaginal and other smears
and cultures for Candida don't
help.**

Therefore the diagnosis†
is suspected from your
history

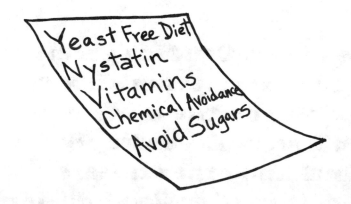

MEDICAL HISTORY

Vaginitis
Athletes Foot
Headaches
Fatigue
Antibiotics
Constipation
etc.

and confirmed by your response
to treatment.

Yeast Free Diet
Nystatin
Vitamins
Chemical Avoidance
Avoid Sugars

---

†Your physician may obtain clues by noting your reponse to testing with Candida extract.

6

Candida Questionnaire And Score Sheet

This questionnaire is designed for adults and the scoring system isn't appropriate for children. It lists factors in your medical history which promote the growth of candida albicans (Section A), and symptoms commonly found in individuals with yeast-connected illness (Section B and C).

For each "Yes" answer in Section A, circle the Point Score in that section. Total your score and record it in the box at the end of the section. Then move on to Sections B and C and score as directed.

Filling out and scoring this questionnaire should help you and your physician evaluate the possible role of candida in contributing to your health problems. Yet it will not provide an automatic "Yes" or "No" answer.

This questionnaire is available in quantity from Professional Books, P.O. Box 3494, Jackson, Tennessee 38301. Prices on request.

Copyright ©, 1983, William G. Crook, M.D.

1. Have you taken tetracyclines (Sumycin®, Panmycin®, Vibramycin®, Minocin®, etc.) or other antibiotics for acne for 1 month (or longer)?	35
2. Have you, at any time in your life, taken other "broad spectrum" antibiotics† for respiratory, urinary or other infections (for 2 months or longer, or in shorter courses 4 or more times in a 1-year period?)	35
3. Have you taken a broad spectrum antibiotic drug†—even a single course?	6
4. Have you, at any time in your life, been bothered by persistent prostatitis, vaginitis or other problems affecting your reproductive organs?	25
5. Have you been pregnant . . .	
2 or more times?	5
1 time?	3
6. Have you taken birth control pills . . .	
For more than 2 years?	15
For 6 months to 2 years?	8
7. Have you taken prednisone, Decadron® or other cortisone-type drugs . . .	
For more than 2 weeks?	15
For 2 weeks or less?	6
8. Does exposure to perfumes, insecticides, fabric shop odors and other chemicals provoke . . .	
Moderate to severe symptoms?	20
Mild symptoms?	5
9. Are your symptoms worse on damp, muggy days or in moldy places?	20
10. Have you had athlete's foot, ring worm, "jock itch" or other chronic fungous infections of the skin or nails? Have such infections been . . .	
Severe or persistent?	20

† Including Keflex,® ampicillin, amoxicillin, Ceclor,® Bactrim® and Septra®. Such antibiotics kill off "good germs" while they're killing off those which cause infection.

Mild to moderate?	—	10
11. Do you crave sugar?	—	10
12. Do you crave breads?		10
13. Do you crave alcoholic beverages?	—	10
14. Does tobacco smoke *really* bother you?	—	10
Total Score, Section A......................		141

SECTION B: MAJOR SYMPTOMS:

For each of your symptoms, enter the appropriate figure in the Point
Score column:

If a symptom is *occasional or mild*...............score 3 points
If a symptom is *frequent and/or moderately severe*.score 6 points
If a symptom is *severe and/or disabling*,..........score 9 points
Add total score and record it in the box at the end of this section.

Point
Score

1. Fatigue or lethargy	6	9
2. Feeling of being "drained"	6	9
3. Poor memory	9	3
4. Feeling "spacey" or "unreal"		3
5. Depression	3	0
6. Numbness, burning or tingling	3	3
7. Muscle aches	3	3
8. Muscle weakness or paralysis		0
9. Pain and/or swelling in joints	3	6
10. Abdominal pain		6
11. Constipation		9
12. Diarrhea		0
13. Bloating	3	3
14. Troublesome vaginal discharge		0
15. Persistent vaginal burning or itching	3	0
16. Prostatitis		
17. Impotence		

31

18. Loss of sexual desire		
19. Endometriosis		6
20. Cramps and/or other menstrual irregularities		
21. Premenstrual tension		
22. Spots in front of eyes		3
23. Erratic vision		3
Total Score, Section B.		51

SECTION C: OTHER SYMPTOMS:†

For each of your symptoms, enter the appropriate figure in the Point Score column:

If a symptom is *occasional or mild*. . . . . .score 1 point
If a symptom is *frequent and/or moderately severe*. score 2 points
If a symptom is *severe and/or disabling,* . . . . .score 3 points
Add total score and record it in the box at the end of this section.

		Point Score
1. Drowsiness		2
2. Irritability or jitteriness	2	1
3. Incoordination	2	0
4. Inability to concentrate	2	2
5. Frequent mood swings		0
6. Headache	1	0
7. Dizziness/loss of balance	1	2
8. Pressure above ears . . . feeling of head swelling & tingling		0
9. Itching	1	1
10. Other rashes		0
11. Heartburn		0
12. Indigestion		3
13. Belching and intestinal gas		3
14. Mucus in stools	1	0

† While the symptoms in this section commonly occur in people with yeast-connected illness they are also found in other individuals.

32

15. Hemorrhoids		2
16. Dry mouth	2	
17. Rash or blisters in mouth		
18. Bad breath	1	3
19. Joint swelling or arthritis	2	
20. Nasal congestion or discharge	1	3
21. Postnasal drip	1	1
22. Nasal itching		2
23. Sore or dry throat		1
24. Cough	1	
25. Pain or tightness in chest	3	
26. Wheezing or shortness of breath	1	
27. Urgency or urinary frequency	1	1
28. Burning on urination	1	1
29. Failing vision		
30. Burning or tearing of eyes	3	
31. Recurrent infections or fluid in ears		
32. Ear pain or deafness		

Total Score, Section C.......................... 25

Total Score, Section A.......................... 54

Total Score, Section B.......................... 141

29
49
96
—
174

GRAND TOTAL SCORE........................... 217

The Grand Total Score will help you and your physician decide if your health problems are yeast-connected. Scores in women will run higher as 7 items in the questionnaire apply exclusively to women, while only 2 apply exclusively to men.

Yeast-connected health problems are almost certainly present in women with scores *over 180,* and in men with scores *over 140.*

Yeast-connected health problems are probably present in women with scores *over 120* and in men with scores *over 90*

Yeast-connected health problems are possibly present in women with scores *over 60* and in men with scores *over 40.*

With scores of less than 60 in women and 40 in men, yeasts are less apt to cause health problems.

7

Treating Your Candida Problem

If I have a Candida problem how do I get rid of it?

you avoid foods which promote yeast growth

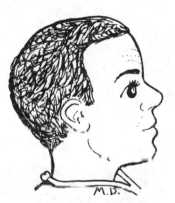

and you take medication which helps rid your body of yeast germs

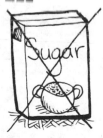

you also need to avoid birth control pills, antibiotics

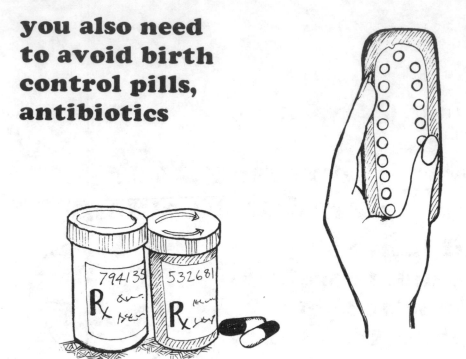

and environmental molds

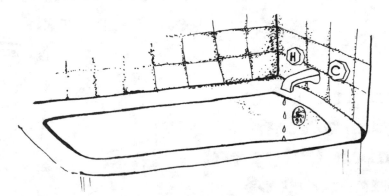

you also need to take other steps to improve your health

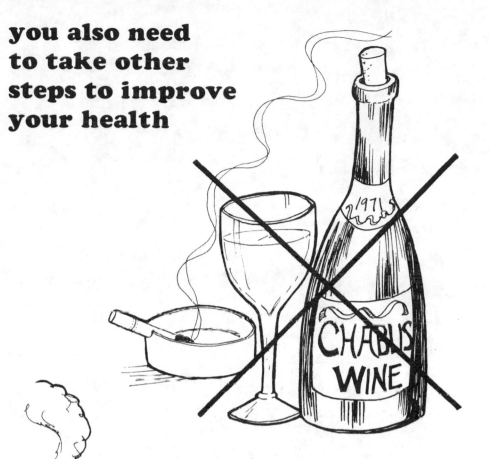

and sometimes your physician may treat you with Candida extract

8

Overcoming Yeast-Connected Illness. . . Questions And Answers

(Q) Tell me more about "The Yeast Connection." And how can you tell if yeasts play a significant role in causing my health problems?

(A) If you're tired and feel bad all over, especially if your fatigue isn't relieved by a night's rest . . .

(Q) That's me. I feel "drained" . . . no matter how much rest I get.

(A) And if you're bothered by all sorts of other peculiar nervous system symptoms . . .

(Q) Like feeling spaced out, jittery and nervous . . . and forgetful? Sometimes I go to the pantry or refrigerator to get something and when I get there I've forgotten what I was looking for . . .

(A) Those are typical symptoms. Here are other symptoms that suggest candida: Problems with digestion, including diarrhea, bloating, gas and constipation.

(Q) Constipation!! I was *never* constipated until the last couple of years. But now, even though I eat tons of prunes and bran, I stay constipated. And gas . . . that's become really embarrassing. What other symptoms? . . .

(A) Those involving your reproductive organs, including severe menstrual cramps, menstrual irregularities and premenstrual tension.

(Q) You mean it could have something to do with me being hard to get along with and feeling like a stuffed sausage the week before my period starts? My husband can't stand me and I can't stand myself.

(A) Yes. And some of my candida patients tell me they gain 3 or 4 pounds during the week before their period and lose it after their period starts.

(Q) Does candida bother only women? I'm wondering if my husband has this problem. He's tired, grumpy and irritable, and is forever treating his jock itch and athlete's foot with powder. He's also visited a urologist because of prostate trouble.

(A) Sounds like he may have the problem too. Recent research by a number of professionals, including Patricia Lucas, Ph.D.[4] suggests that candida *is* a low grade infection which can be transmitted by close association. Moreover, your husband's symptoms certainly suggest that he could have the problem, too.

(Q) OK . . . , you suspect the candida problem from my history. How do you go about making a positive diagnosis . . . do tests help?

(A) No . . . or not much. Here's why: Candida germs are present in everyone's body . . . yours included. They live on your mucous membranes, in your digestive tract† and in your vagina, even if you aren't troubled by digestive symptoms or vaginitis. Accordingly, smears and cultures which show candida don't help.

(Q) If tests don't help, what do you do? How can you make a positive diagnosis of a candida problem? Or how can you rule it out?

(A) If a careful history, physical examination and appropriate diagnostic tests and studies rule out other causes for your symptoms, I prescribe an anticandida treatment program and note your response. I call this a "therapeutic trial."

---

† Research studies to determine the level of candida in the stool are now being carried out in several medical centers. Perhaps objective laboratory data which will help in the diagnosis of the patient with candida-related illness may be available in the near future.

(Q) "Therapeutic trial?" . . . Tell me more about it . . . What does it consist of?

(A) It's a treatment program designed to *discourage* the growth of candida germs in your body, especially in your digestive tract and in your vagina.

(A) The program consists of two main parts . . . a special diet† and nystatin or other anti-yeast medication. Let's talk about your diet first.

You'll need to eat foods that do *not* encourage the growth of yeasts in your digestive system. Feature high protein foods, including fish, seafood, nuts and eggs. Try to fill up on vegetables, especially the low-carbohydrate vegetables, including lettuce, spinach, broccoli, squash, cauliflower, cucumbers and asparagus. Avoid white flour, refined grain products, and avoid or limit fruits (see also pages 117-120).

(Q) What foods should I avoid?

(A) Candies, cakes, ice cream, soft drinks and sugar-containing foods of all sorts. Also honey, maple syrup and carob.

(Q) No way! I'm a sugar addict. I can't live without sweets.

(A) I'm not surprised. Sugar craving occurs commonly in people with the candida problem. So what you're saying makes me suspect candida even more.

(Q) How about fructose, and honey, and corn syrup? Are they as bad as ordinary table sugar?

(A) Yes. Just as bad, and they encourage the growth of yeasts , like rain makes grass, weeds and mushrooms grow.

(Q) What foods besides sweets should I avoid?

(A) Most breads and bakery products . . . since they contain yeast . . . and other foods and beverages which contain yeast.

---

† For a detailed discussion of dietary factors, see pages 67-125.

(Q) What are some of them?

(A) Wine, beer and all alcoholic and fermented beverages. Read labels and stay away from anything that contains malt. You'll also need to avoid mushrooms, all cheeses, vinegar, dried fruits and melons, especially cantaloupe.

(Q) Are there other sources of yeast I need to know about?

(A) Yes. Since many or most antibiotics are derived from molds, don't take antibiotics unless you really need them. Then there are vitamins.

(Q) What about vitamins?

(A) Many vitamins, especially members of the B-complex, are derived from yeast. So if you're taking a vitamin, make sure the label specifies "no yeast."

(Q) Let's talk more about "carbohydrates" since I've heard they promote the growth of the yeast germ. How much carbohydrate can I eat?

(A) It will depend on the severity and duration of your symptoms. Usually, I tell my patients, "The amount of carbohydrate you can tolerate (like the dose of nystatin) must be determined by trial and error.

Many of my patients seem to tolerate all of the 'good carbohydrates' found in vegetables, whole grains and fruits unless they're allergic to these foods. However, at the recently concluded Birmingham conference on *Human—Yeast Interaction* (December, 1983), John W. Rippon, Ph.D., an authority on yeast and molds said, "Fruits and sugars promote yeast growth, while vegetables and whole grains do not." (see also pages 67-73, 94-110, 119-120.) Because of its high content of the simple carbohydrate lactose, milk also promotes yeast growth. (For further comments on milk, see pages 100, 293-294.)

(Q) We've talked about my husband. Now I'd like to talk about my children. My 6-year-old son is hyperactive and keeps a cold and has been given numerous rounds of antibiotics. And my year old baby is experiencing all sorts of health problems. One cold after another, five ear infections, and a month ago tubes were put in his ears. His nose stays congested and he's irritable and restless. Do you think the anti-candida program will help them?

(A) Yes. Although I've treated more adults than children with candida-related illness during the past year, I've found that candida plays an important role in causing health problems in many of my pediatric patients. (See pages 195-211.)

Naturally, before putting your children on an anti-candida treatment program, I need to examine them and carefully review their histories, because factors other than candida can play a role in causing the health problems you describe. For example, inhalant allergies, hidden food allergies and nutritional deficiencies may contribute to health disorders in children of all ages.

(Q) Suppose they were put on the anti-candida program. What sort of diet restrictions would you recommend?

(A) I restrict sugar and other refined carbohydrates in all of my pediatric patients, even those in whom I don't suspect candida. My own observations,[5-a,b,c] as well as those of Cheraskin,[6] Prinz[7] and others[8-a,b,c] make me feel that sugar may bother both children and adults. Such individuals tend to develop emotional and behavior problems and suffer from recurrent respiratory infections. So keep your children off sugar and corn syrup, and go easy on the honey. *Do not limit their good complex carbohydrates.* Offer them a variety of nutritious foods, including meats, eggs, vegetables, whole grains, nuts, seeds, fresh fruits†and some dairy products, if they aren't allergic to milk.

In infants still taking a formula, I prescribe a special soy formula which contains no corn syrup or other refined carbohydrates. And I use cereal grains, fruits‡ and vegetables to supply the child's carbohydrate needs. (See pages 209-210.)

Avoid juices, especially those which are canned or frozen, because nearly all contain yeast. However, you could get oranges, squeeze them and prepare fresh juice‡.

Make or buy some specially-prepared yeast-free breads and crackers, since the usual bakery products contain molds and yeast, as well as sugar. (See pages 86, 115-117.)

---

‡ Based on the research studies of Rippon and Odds, fruits may also need to be limited (see pages 73, 119-120.)

(Q) OK. Back to my own situation. Other than following the diet, what else should I do?

(A) You'll need a medication which helps eradicate or control the yeast organisms in your digestive tract. Nystatin is the medication I usually prescribe for my patients with yeast-connected health problems.

(Q) What kind of medicine is nystatin?

(A) Nystatin is an anti-fungal drug which kills yeasts and yeast-like fungi. Yet it doesn't affect bacteria and other germs.

(Q) What form does nystatin come in? Is it available on prescription?

(A) Nystatin is available on prescription in 500,000 unit oral tablets. These tablets are marketed by Lederle under the brand name Nilstat® and by Squibb under the brand name Mycostatin®. Nystatin is also available in liquid oral suspensions, vaginal tablets and suppositories,† and topical powders. Generic preparations of nystatin are also available.

Still another form, chemically-pure nystatin powder, is manufactured by The American Cyanamid Company, Lederle division. Pharmacists, hospitals, clinics and physicians can obtain information about nystatin powder by calling 1-800-LEDERLE.††

(Q) Does nystatin often cause adverse reactions . . . or side effects?

(A) Nystatin is an unusually safe medicine . . . as safe or safer than most drugs physicians prescribe for their patients. According to the *Physician's Desk Reference*[9] (which gives information on over 2500 prescription drugs), "Nystatin is virtually non-toxic and non-sensitizing and is well tolerated by all age groups, even on prolonged administration."

Here's a major reason for the safety of nystatin . . . *very little is*

---

† Women with yeast-connected health problems should take appropriate steps to control candida in the vagina—*even if they are NOT bothered by vaginal symptoms*. Effective preparations include Mycelex G®, Monistat-7® and Gyne-Lotrimin® creams and suppositories. Yogurt douches are also effective as are intravaginal preparations of nystatin. (See also page 247).

†† A word of caution about nystatin powder: Most pharmacists stock a Mycostatin Topical Powder® (Squibb). This powder is prepared for use on the skin and is not to be confused with the pure nystatin powder.

absorbed from the intestinal tract. Accordingly, it helps the person with yeast-related health problems by killing candida in the digestive tract.

Nevertheless, it disagrees with some patients and may cause digestive symptoms or skin rashes. In addition, some individuals develop other symptoms, including headache, fatigue and flu-like symptoms, especially during the first few days of treatment. Fortunately, these symptoms usually subside within several days, even though the medication is continued.

(Q) What causes these symptoms? Do they develop because of an allergy to the nystatin?

(A) Although scientists haven't yet determined the mechanism of these reactions, many experts believe they occur when your body absorbs large quantities of killed yeast germs. Somewhat similar reactions to the killing off of other harmful micro-organisms were first described almost 100 years ago and are sometimes referred to as "Herxheimer" reactions.

A physician consultant who has suffered from candida-related illness commented, "As long as nystatin causes symptoms, it's probably killing candida. And in my experience, most patients who develop such symptoms can take nystatin at a reduced dose, if symptoms are intolerable. Then, as they improve, they can usually take larger doses." (See also page 249.)

(Q) Could reactions to nystatin make it necessary for me to stop the drug or change the dose?

(A) Yes, but before I give up on nystatin, I instruct my patients to experiment with the dose, as the proper dose of nystatin must be determined by trial and error. Moreover, the correct dose varies from patient to patient.

Most of my patients improve when they take 500,000 to 1,000,000 units (1 or 2 tablets or 1/8 to 1/4 teaspoon of the powder) of nystatin four times a day. However, some patients require 4 to 8 tablets or 1/2 to 1 teaspoon of the powder four times a day. And a rare patient requires an even larger dose. By contrast, an occasional patient does well on a dose of 1/16 teaspoonful (or less) given 4 times a day.

Now, I'd like to repeat and clarify my comments about reactions.

Many of my patients show a temporary worsening of symptoms after starting to take nystatin.

Such symptoms aren't normally caused by an allergic reaction to the nystatin. Instead, they indicate that the nystatin is killing the candida and the patient may need either a bigger dose or a smaller dose. Symptoms of too big a dose include flushing, fever and flu-like symptoms. By contrast, fatigue, headache, depression and digestive upsets are common underdose symptoms that will often improve on a bigger dose. Either type of reaction usually subsides in 4 to 7 days, even though the medication is continued.

An occasional patient has developed more severe symptoms, including severe headaches, depression, fatigue, muscle aching, vomiting, diarrhea or skin rashes. Usually, these symptoms occur during the early days or weeks of nystatin treatment. However, such reactions may rarely occur in patients who have been taking nystatin for several months without previous adverse side effects.

When nystatin reactions persist, I may recommend that the patient discontinue the medication for 2 to 3 weeks. Then, following the recommendation of Dr. Phyllis Saifer of Berkeley, California, I sometimes try it again in tiny amounts . . . Dr. Saifer calls them "dot doses."

(Q) Just what is a "dot dose"?†

(A) A "dot" is the amount you can pick up on the flat end of a toothpick. In using this dose, I give a patient these instructions:

"Take 1 'dot' the first day. Then if you tolerate this dose and show no side-effects, in 48 hours take one 'dot' twice a day.

If you tolerate two 'dots' a day, after another 48 hours, try three 'dots' a day. Cautiously increase your dose of nystatin until you improve or develop unpleasant side-effects. If you tolerate gradually increasing doses of nystatin, build up your dose to 1/8 to 1/2 teaspoon four times a day in 2 to 4 weeks." "*Your exact dose will depend on your response.*"

---

†Over a period of several months, I started many patients on "dot" doses and I noted more adverse reactions to nystatin than I had noted in patients who started treatment with larger doses. So I now start most of my patients on 1/8 to 1/4 teaspoon (or one or two 500,000 unit tablets) four times a day.

(Q) If nystatin powder disagrees with me and causes side-effects, could I use the nystatin tablets? They'd be more convenient and easier to take.

(A) Although nystatin tablets agree with most patients, I usually recommend nystatin powder. Here's why:

1. Yeast organisms live in your digestive tract, from your mouth to your rectum. Accordingly, the powder helps you get rid of yeast in the upper part of the digestive tract, as well as in your intestines.

2. The powder contains no food coloring, chemicals, dye or other similar ingredients which may cause reactions in chemically-sensitive patients.

3. The powder is more economical.

(Q) Do precautions need to be taken in handling and storing the powder?

(A) Yes. The powder should be refrigerated. In talking to a representative from the manufacturer, she commented, "We ship the powder through ordinary channels and it does not lose significant potency in several days without refrigeration. However, potency is more apt to be retained when the powder is refrigerated."

(Q) How should I take the powder?

(A) Here's a method used by many physicians: Add the prescribed dose to 2 or 3 ounces of water, then take a large mouthful and swish it around for a minute or so before swallowing. Then drink the rest of the dose.

Here's another way I like better. Dump the nystatin powder on your tongue and let it gradually dissolve in your mouth. I prefer this method and feel it is more effective. I realize the powder has a bitter taste, but not as bitter as many other medicines. Moreover, the taste soon goes away.

Some of my patients say, "At work or especially when I'm traveling, I find it inconvenient or impossible to take nystatin powder during the day. So I like the tablets during the day and the powder for my morning and evening doses."

(Q) Are dye-free tablets or capsules of nystatin available that I could use in place of the powder for my daytime dose of nystatin?

(A) Although dye-free tablets aren't manufactured by the large pharmaceutical firms, some pharmacists prepare and dispense nystatin powder in dye-free capsules.

(Q) If nystatin helps me, how long will I need to take it?

(A) This will depend on your response. You'll need to take it for many, many months . . . or until you're well. And some of my patients have required nystatin for a year or longer. Try to be patient.

(Q) Suppose the nystatin disagrees with me, or suppose my symptoms continue to bother me. Is there a medication other than nystatin which can be used?

(A) Yes . . . ketoconazole . . . a drug which has been used extensively in Europe for a number of years without serious reactions. Ketoconazole was first licensed by the Federal Drug Administration (FDA) in August, 1981 for use in treating fungal infections. It is now marketed in this country by the Janssen Company under the name Nizoral®.

Nizoral® is a potent, valuable drug. And in certain ways it is superior to nystatin. Like many effective medications, it is absorbed from the intestinal tract and transported by the circulation to various parts of the body. So it not only kills yeast germs in your digestive tract, it also helps eradicate them in your vagina, skin and other tissues of your body.

(Q) Why don't you prescribe Nizoral® for all of your patients with the candida problem?

(A) Because Nizoral® may rarely cause side-effects, more especially liver inflammation. According to a recent report by the FDA, "Serious liver injury was not observed in clinical trials before the drug's approval for marketing in the United States. It became manifest only when large numbers of persons began taking the drug."

During the first year of its use in the United States, approximately 150,000 prescriptions for Nizoral® were written. Three deaths have been reported in patients who had been taking Nizoral®. However, these patients had severe, life-threatening disorders before the Nizoral® was started. The FDA received reports of 20 additional patients who showed signs of minor liver irritation.

(Q) Let's talk more about Nizoral® . Since it causes such side-effects, is it worth the risk? And what can be done to lessen the risk?

(A) Everything you do carries a risk. And fatal reactions have occurred from aspirin, penicillin and other drugs you've taken. In spite of the possible side effects of Nizoral®, many physicians prescribe it for their patients with candida-related health problems.

In discussing the side-effects and risks of Nizoral®, the warning section on the label, prepared by the manufacturer, states, "It's important to perform liver function tests . . . before treatment and at periodic intervals during treatment (monthly or more frequently), particularly in patients who will be on prolonged therapy or who have a history of liver disease."

(Q) Do you prescribe Nizoral® for your patients? Or more specifically, would you prescribe it for me?

(A) Yes, especially if you didn't improve on nystatin or if you did not tolerate nystatin. However, before giving up on nystatin, I usually have my patients increase their dose to 1 teaspoon of the powder four times a day. And I occasionally prescribe even larger doses.

(Q) Gosh, that seems like a lot. Why would I need that much nystatin?

(A) Such a big dose of nystatin will enable your body to absorb enough nystatin to get in the blood stream and reach yeast germs which may have invaded the deeper layers of your mucous membranes. And by reaching and killing off such organisms, improvement may occur which did not take place on the smaller dose.

I also remind my patients that candida isn't "the cause" of their health problems and that nystatin . . . as helpful as it is . . . isn't a magic bullet that will cure them. And I repeatedly stress other treatment measures that are important (these are described in Section C, pages 131-175.)

Also, before giving up on nystatin, I usually have my patients experiment further with their diets. As I've already pointed out, I recommend the Low Carbohydrate Diet when a patient doesn't improve on the Candida Control Diet. Moreover, in some patients, I look for adverse or allergic reactions to foods, including foods other than carbohydrates. I try such patients on what I've termed the "cave man diet." (See page 129.)

(Q) And if these various measures didn't work, you'd try the Nizoral® ?

(A) Yes. And occasionally I prescribe Nizoral® even before I use nystatin. Nizoral® has helped dozens of my patients and none of them has experienced significant side effects from the drug. Moreover, after a patient improves on Nizoral®, the dose can usually be reduced without causing a flareup in symptoms. And in some, I've found I could substitute nystatin for Nizoral® after a few weeks of treatment.

I'd like to stress again that *each person is different*, and I try to tailor treatment programs so that they fit the unique needs of each patient.

(Q) I'd like to get more information about the anti-candida medicines. I'm particularly interested in the relative costs of nystatin and Nizoral®. And is cost a consideration?

(A) Yes, at times it is. The cost of nystatin will be significantly greater than the cost of Nizoral® when it is taken in large doses. So I consider the seriousness of a patient's disorder and the cost of the medication, as well as the risks involved, in deciding which medicine to use. *Yet, nystatin remains the safest and best medication for most of my patients and it's the one I usually prescribe.*

(Q) Are there other drugs which help kill out candida?

(A) Yes. Clotrimazole and amphotericin B. However, the latter drug isn't available in the United States in an oral preparation except in combination with tetracycline. (See pages 256, 279-83 for additional comments on these drugs).

50

(Q) What else will I need to do to overcome the yeast problem and regain my health?

(A) Molds and yeast are kin to each other. So you should lessen your exposure to molds in any and every way you can, both at home and in your work-place. Here's why: Molds you breathe can trigger your symptoms.

(Q) What can I do to avoid molds and get rid of them?

(A) Learn as much as you can about where molds are found and take steps to avoid them.

Common sources of airborne molds include bathrooms, damp basements, carpeting, poorly ventilated closets, old upholstered furniture, humidifiers, decaying leaves, stored fruits and vegetables, old wallpaper and home air ducts. (See pages 55-64 for a discussion of the effects of environmental molds.)

(Q) I've read and heard about yeast vaccines. Could such a vaccine help me?

(A) Possibly. In some of my patients, the yeast vaccine has worked like a miracle in relieving symptoms. Apparently it helps by stimulating the immune system. Yet, the vaccine disagrees with many of the patients.

In my own practice, I sometimes use the vaccine and sometimes I don't. In your case, I'm going to wait and try you on the other treatment measures we've talked about. Then, depending on your response, we may use the vaccine later on. (For further discussion on the use of candida extracts or vaccines in diagnosis and treatment, see pages 252-254.)

(Q) What else do I need to do?

(A) Many things. Here's why: When you're sick or don't feel well, your health problems are nearly always due to a variety of causes rather than a single one. And although taking anti-candida medication and avoiding sugar and yeast containing foods will help you regain your health, you'll also need to pay attention to many other factors. (A more complete discussion of some of the causes of illness can be found in Section C.)

You are what you eat. And you need to eat a variety of wholesome foods, including proteins, complex carbohydrates and essential fats and oils. I also prescribe nutritional supplements, including vitamins and minerals. You must also avoid poisons and pollutants of all kinds, including those which contaminate the air, soil and water; and you must limit your intake of nutritionally-poor food, including sugar, white flour and hardened vegetable oil.

If you're troubled by allergies to food and inhalants, these must be properly treated. You also need a favorable environment, including fresh air, sunlight, pure water and the loving support of those around you.

A few final words: Although I'm certain your health disorder is yeast connected, what we'll be treating is your immune system and not just the yeast germ, *Candida albicans.* So be patient. Your health problems didn't develop overnight and they won't go away in a few days or a few weeks or months. Yet, if you're like most of my patients with yeast-connected health problems, be of good cheer! *You will get well.*

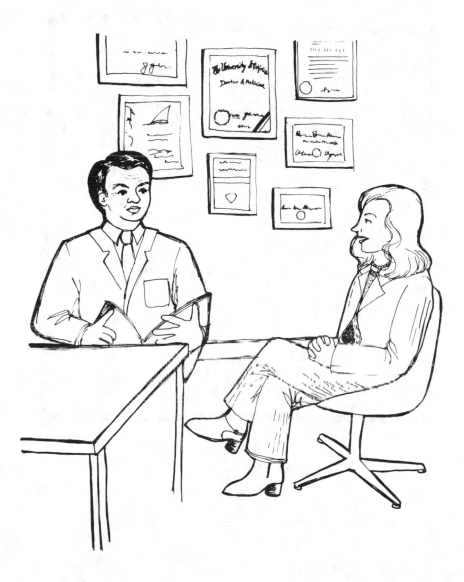

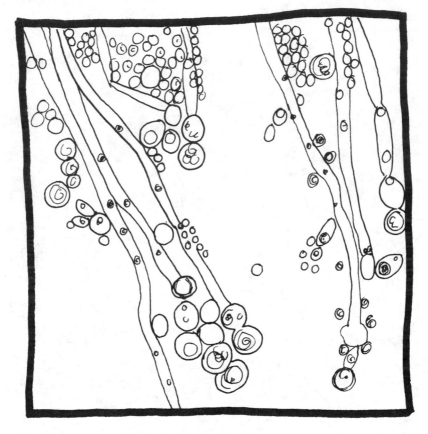

Mold hyphae and spores
(microscopic view)

9

More About Yeasts, Molds And Other Fungi

If candida plays a role in making you sick, eating or breathing other yeasts and molds will aggravate your symptoms. So you should learn about yeasts and molds and take steps to avoid them. (See also pages 2-4.)

Yeasts and molds are members of the vegetable kingdom. Generally speaking, yeasts are oval or elliptical single-celled organisms. By contrast, molds form colonies and each cell grows long, intertwining, hair-like branches called "hyphae."

However, identifying a particular yeast or mold isn't easy. Here's why: Sometimes these little plants can change from a mold to a yeast, and back again.

Yeast and molds live all around us. They commonly grow on fruits and vegetables, especially dried fruits and grapes. They're also found in the soil, air and water. Some outdoor molds die when snow covers the ground. Yet, even in the wintertime, mold spores live in the soil.

Mold spores float in the air like pollen. So you can breathe them and they may be deposited in your lungs, as well as in your nose and throat.

Some molds are found on decomposing plants, leather, cloth, rubber, wood and paper products. Others grow outdoors on vegetation.

Conditions that promote mold growth can be summarized in two words: *Dampness* and *darkness*. Accordingly, if you want to control molds around you, change the conditions that favor their growth. Sometimes you can accomplish this by using a dehumidifier, especially in damp basements or closets. You can also destroy molds by applying a boric solution. A low-wattage bulb burning in a closet will lessen the mold population. And an electric heat lamp designed to dry out dark closets is available from the Damp Chaser Electronics, Inc., Hendersonville, N.C. 28739.

If you're sensitive to molds, get rid of the mold catchers in your home. And there are many of these, including old books, upholstered furniture and flower pots. Washing, airing and sunning will help retard mold growth on your bed clothing, pillows, mattress pads and rugs.

Besides candida and air-borne molds, other yeasts and fungi are found in foods you eat every day. Among the more obvious of these foods are mushrooms, aged cheeses and alcoholic beverages. Yeasts are also found in fermented beverages and in baked goods that rise. They also grow quickly in fruit juices and foods that ferment easily. (See also page 89.)

Yeast growth in your body is also encouraged or stimulated by medications of various types, including especially antibiotics, birth control pills and the corticosteroid group of drugs.

Sources Of Mold In Homes

Damp basements — especially those with dirt floors — encourage mold growth. (Moisture tends to evaporate from the floor; this draws additional soil water into the house by capillary action.)

Bathrooms provide a comfortable home for molds. They love every nook, and cranny. They'll grow in your bath tub drain and on wash cloths, damp towels, crevices or cracks in the wall covering.

Closets, drawers or hampers often promote mold growth, especially when you load them up with clothing you've worn that hasn't been laundered. (Perspiration encourages mold growth as do shoes saturated with perspiration.)

Mattresses and other bedding sometimes become mold infested. Mold growth can be lessened by washing the mattress pads frequently.

Carpets of all kinds encourage mold growth, especially shag carpets. You can lessen mold exposure by using throw rugs. (Wash them often!)

Old upholstered furniture, bedding, pillows, rags, sleeping bags or other items, particularly those made from natural fibers.

Old newspapers, books or magazines.

Flower pots and dried or decaying plant materials.

Houses, especially those in shaded areas or near rivers or streams, tend to collect mold. Shrubs or vines planted close to your house retain moisture and tend to encourage mold growth.

Humidifers, especially vaporizers, encourage mold growth.

Kitchens that are inadequately ventilated. The area between the kitchen sink and the wall, around the bottom of the cold water pipe, wood chopping boards marred from use and rotting fruits and vegetables are all locations molds favor. Other sites include the rubber gasket that seals the refrigerator door and the surplus water tray located in the bottom of self-defrosting refrigerators.

Decaying leaves, compost, lawn clippings or hay. Raking or mowing the grass launches millions of mold spores and fragments into the air.

Some wallpapers contain chemical mold-retardants. However, these chemicals may "outgas" and cause symptoms in some chemically sensitive individuals.

Fruits or vegetables stored in a basement or cellar. Potatoes, carrots and other root vegetables begin to mold soon after they're taken from the ground.

Controlling Yeasts And Molds

Avoid molds at home and at work

One of my patients with severe health problems related to candida was improving on a treatment program which included nystatin and a low-carbohydrate, yeast-free diet. At one of her recheck visits, she came in with this story:

> "I knew I felt worse in damp weather or when I went to my moldy basement. I also noted that if I worked in the kitchen for more than a few minutes, I would develop a headache and feel 'spaced out' and depressed. So with my husband's help, I did some detective work. We found heavy mold growth under the sink. My husband cleaned it out and now the kitchen doesn't bother me."

Another patient, a physician, suffered from severe, incapacitating depression. Many mornings he found it impossible to get out of bed or to carry out any useful work. Although he realized that going to the basement or other moldy places aggravated his symptoms, he had not associated his severe symptoms with molds in his home.

Then he was hospitalized because of a bleeding ulcer. Even though he was seriously ill and four pints of blood were necessary for therapy, he was amazed to find that while in the hospital his fatigue and depression vanished. He commented,

> "I felt better than I had felt since I played football in college . . . lots of energy, no depression, and I was able to think clearly."

Following recovery, he returned to his home and, within 2 to 3 days, his symptoms of fatigue and depression returned. When he stayed out of his home for 3 days on a trip, his symptoms disappeared.

On testing with candida extract, his symptoms of depression and mental dullness were provoked by the initial test dose and blocked or neutralized when he was given a different dose.

One of my patients was interviewed recently by Mary Reed, Features Editor of *The Jackson Sun*. In a special article on yeast-connected health problems, published on May 26, 1983, Mary wrote:

> "Marilyn Smith's problems started about 15 years ago when she started taking birth control pills, but they really got bad after her third child was born four years ago. The problem progressed over the years until Marilyn thought she was having a nervous breakdown.
>
> "Besides having joint swelling and other arthritic symptoms, Mrs. Smith would become emotional, get migraine headaches, get dizzy and faint. Her colon and stomach would hurt so much she could hardly walk.
>
> "Marilyn commented, 'I've cried for days and days at a time. My family thought I was losing my mind. It's just horrid.'
>
> "Today, she knows her allergies to yeast and some other foods were the cause of her problems. If she eats white potatoes, she'll get a headache almost immediately. Like other patients, *even smelling yeast or mold brings on symptoms*. Recently, she walked into a school cafeteria where yeast cinnamon rolls were baking and she just started crying.
>
> "Now that she avoids yeast-containing foods, processed sugar and places like bakeries and greenhouses (which have a lot of mold in the air), Marilyn's life has changed. 'When I found out I wasn't crazy, it was so wonderful'."

Three of my patients work at the local office of the Social Security Administration and are bothered by many candida-related symptoms. Recently, one of them commented,

"The office I work in makes me sick. It's full of mold. The roof leaked last year and the whole building is damp. We've even found mold growing on records in the filing cabinet. I feel much better on weekends when I'm at home. Then when I go back to the office my symptoms return."

Two of my patients who work in a restaurant featuring pizza noted their symptoms gradually became worse while working there. On weekends off or vacation, symptoms would improve.

If your home or work place is loaded with molds, your yeast-connected health problems may bother you until you take measures to lessen your exposure to molds (see pages 61-64.) And you may even need to change jobs or find another place to live.

Avoid antibiotics

If you develop a "strep throat," pneumonia, meningitis or a kidney infection, you'll need to be treated with an antibiotic drug to help your body combat the invading bacteria. But if you do not have such a disorder (even if you run a fever), chances are you don't need such medication. If you're bothered by yeast-related illness, take antibiotics only when absolutely necessary, since antibiotics promote the growth of the yeast germ in your body.

Some 80 to 90 percent of respiratory infections are caused by viruses and such illnesses aren't helped by antibiotics. So if you come down with a fever, cough or cold, don't pressure your physician to give you an antibiotic unless he finds it essential.

When antibiotics are necessary, I usually prescribe penicillin G, penicillin V or erythromycin rather then Keflex®, Ceclor®, ampicillin, amoxicillin, Septra®, Bactrim®, or other "broad-spectrum" antibiotics. Here's why: penicillin and erythromycin attack mainly the "strep" and pneumonia germs found in the nose, throat and lungs. (However, they, too, may activate either vaginal or digestive tract yeast.) By contrast, the broad-spectrum drugs kill these same organisms and also destroy many normal intestinal and vaginal bacteria. And when such bacteria are wiped out, yeast germs are more apt to take their place.

I also usually prescribe nystatin along with the antibiotic. Nystatin is, of course, indicated in patients with immune system problems related to candida. However, even in patients in whom such a relationship is uncertain, especially children with recurrent ear infections, I prescribe nystatin along with the antibiotic. And I discontinue the antibiotic drug as soon as is feasible, depending on the type and duration of the infection.

How about patients who develop infections of the kidney or bladder which require that an antibiotic drug be used in treatment? In discussing such drugs, several urologists have commented, "Most urinary tract infections will respond to the nitrofurantoin drugs, Furadantin® and Macrodantin®. These drugs do not promote the growth of yeast germs." (For a more detailed discussion of these drugs, see pages 200-201.)

I feel that antibiotics are often used when they aren't needed in the treatment of women with urinary tract symptoms. Because such individuals complain of painful and frequent urination, both the physician and the patient assumes the symptoms are caused by cystitis . . . a bacterial infection.

In patients of this type, the symptoms may be due to the generalized candida infection in the vulvovaginal area, giving rise to urethritis. And the use of antibiotic drugs in this condition serves only to aggravate further the yeast infection that is the actual cause of the discomfort.

I've also seen a number of patients with severe yeast-related illness who give a history of taking daily doses of sulfonamide or other antibacterial drugs for months or years to prevent recurrent urinary tract (or ear) infections. Although such drugs may suppress the germs which cause these infections, they also encourage the growth of candida. And the resulting health problems are often worse than those the anti-bacterial drugs were used to prevent. (See, also, pages 222-223.)

I also take a dim view of the long-term use of tetracyclines for acne because I've seen so many patients with severe yeast-connected illness who gave a history of such a treatment program.

Avoid "the pill"

Hormone pills containing both estrogens and progesterone have been widely used during the past two decades for contraception. They are also used commonly in treating women with menstrual cramps and a variety of menstrual irregularities. *Avoidance of the birth control pill is mandatory if chronic candidiasis is to be successfully controlled.*

The progesterone component of these pills causes changes in the vaginal mucous membrane which makes it easier for ever-present yeasts to multiply and cause not only vaginitis, but associated systemic symptoms, including irritability, fatigue and depression. Other mechanisms may also be involved in producing these symptoms, including changes in hormonal function.

Pure estrogen pills which are frequently prescribed for women during and after menopause do not encourage the growth of yeasts.

Treat your home with formaldehyde vapors?

One of my patients (I'll call her Susan) commented,

> "I'm sensitive to all sorts of chemicals. Yet, mold exposure causes severe symptoms, including depression and fatigue. My house is killing me and I can't afford to move. What can I do?"

Getting rid of molds isn't easy. Yet, there are steps which are effective. One of these is the use of formaldehyde, a substance which causes both toxic and allergic reactions in many people, including individuals with yeast-connected illness.

So in discussing this problem with Susan, I said,

> "Anything you do carries a risk, whether it's eating, taking a bath or driving your car to your office. And before making a decision about what you should and should not do, you should weigh the relative risks. And in your situation, I feel you may wish to consider the formaldehyde method of Dr. Marshall Mandell to eliminate molds from your home."

In his book, *Dr. Mandell's 5-day Allergy Relief System,*[10] in a section entitled, "Steps To Take If Mold Is A Problem," Dr. Mandell commented,

> "One day a friend and I were talking about his sailboat. He said, 'You know, whenever I go sailing, I develop a terrible cough which is much worse when I'm down in the cabin'."

Dr. Mandell then told of inspecting the boat and being "overwhelmed" by the musty odor characteristic of mildew (molds). The problem was how to remove the molds for a reasonable period of time without causing a persistent chemical problem from the use of mold-killing agents.

Dr. Mandell described a method suggested by mold allergy expert, Dr. Nathan Schaeffer, using formaldehyde. Using this method was

61

"highly successful" and the boat was completely free of mold; the beneficial effects of the formaldehyde disinfection lasted for approximately two months.

In a letter to me dated April 29, 1983, Dr. Mandell commented,

> "This form of treatment is easily applied to single rooms, basements and entire homes. However, it is necessary for members of the household to remain away from home for a long weekend and arrange to have the house well aired before it is occupied again.
>
> "The average size basement requires from four to six coffee containers (or soup plates or pie pans) with an inch of formaldehyde in the bottom of each. Place one can in each 12' x 12' to 15' x 15' foot area in mold contaminated spaces. This is usually the basement because flooding and condensation occur in the basement area and mold grows on books, papers, carpets, shoes and old clothing. It also grows in dirt crawl spaces and will travel up the cellar stairs and enter the rest of the house.
>
> "However, mold is also encountered in homes with no basements which are constructed on concrete slabs. The slabs are in direct contact with the earth which is always cooler than moisture-laden air of summer and condensation of water may occur on the slab. This may keep carpeting and carpet pads moist and promote mold growth.
>
> "When the entire house seems to be loaded with mold, containers of formaldehyde solution should be put in a number of locations throughout the home, including the basement and attic. Windows should be closed and the home should not be entered for at least two full days.
>
> "Air the house thoroughly when you return or have this done for you and do not re-enter your home until there is no detectable odor of formaldehyde. The airing-out process can be hastened by using electric fans and by swinging several doors back and forth on their hinges, being careful not to be exposed to the fumes."

Formaldehyde in water is available at most drug stores in a one-pound (pint), 37% solution. The formaldehyde/water mixture is referred to as *formalin*; methyl alcohol is added as a sterilizing agent. Mold-killing formaldehyde vapors fill the indoor air as they evaporate from the formalin solution.

In carrying out formaldehyde sterilization/fumigation, the individual pouring the solution into the containers must be protected. Protective goggles are helpful. The individual performing the sterilization should pour the formaldehyde into the container in the most distant or inaccessible part of the basement (farthest away from the door), while holding his/her breath. Then he/she should go outdoors or to an area of the house that's far enough away from the formalin-containing cans so that there is no formaldehyde pollution of the surrounding air. Then he/she should take a deep breath and then fill the next two containers that are closer to the exit. This procedure can be repeated until all containers are filled.

In commenting further on the formaldehyde treatment, Dr. Mandell said in effect,

> "Airing-out of the house with complete elimination of formaldehyde fumes takes from 1/2 to 2 or 3 days, depending on the effectiveness of the airing-out process. It is most unusual to have residual odors after 3 to 5 days. As far as I can tell, formaldehyde fumes do not cling to or "lock into" any substances or material, and in most instances the odor dissipates rapidly."

In his continuing discussion, Dr. Mandell commented, saying in effect,

> "Some ecologically-oriented people have objected to the use of formaldehyde since allergy prone individuals can become sensitized to this reactive substance and suffer adverse effects from formaldehyde exposure. Prolonged formaldehyde exposure in a home can have serious, long-term effects on the health of those who've been exposed. Moreover, it may affect the person's overall resistance to a wide variety of allergens.
> "In my experience, alternative methods for controlling indoor molds, including sodium bicarbonate solutions or aqueous Zephiran®, haven't worked. Here's why: Molds colonize structural areas of the home or building that are completely inaccessible to surface scrubbing. So the only way to treat these areas is to have the anti-fungal material reach them in a vapor state through the evaporation of formaldehyde which is dispersed throughout the atmosphere of the formaldehyde-treated areas of the home. A disinfecting program will be unsatisfactory if all the nooks and crannies are not reached."

In concluding my discussion with Susan, I presented her with the following options:

1. Move out of your moldy house if you can. Even though you feel you can't afford to move, it's something you should consider.
2. Mold cultures and colony counts can be obtained from different rooms in your home. (Information about such studies can be obtained from Mould Service, c/o Sherry A. Rogers, M.D., 2800 West Genesee Street, Syracuse, New York 13219, and from Hollister-Stier Laboratories, P.O. Box 19957, Atlanta, Ga. 30325.)
3. If the mold counts are high, spend a night or two away from your home in a room which is less apt to be contaminated

with molds or chemicals, and see if you can notice a difference.

4. Allergy testing, followed by treatment with mold extracts may help lessen your sensitivity.

5. Get a knowledgeable carpenter or building contractor to take a look at your home and see if he can recommend structural changes which can prevent moisture and prohibit or significantly reduce mold growth, since, as Dr. Mandell pointed out, "The formaldehyde treatment isn't a proper solution for what will be a recurrent problem."

6. Try Dr. Mandell's formaldehyde treatment program. *However, because so many individuals are made ill by formaldehyde and other chemical exposures, I have mixed feelings about recommending this program.* Yet, if you can't move and nothing else helps, and you can get someone else to do the work, you may want to consider it.

Section
B

To control Candida,
you must
change your diet.

10

Introduction

To obtain adequate nutrition, you need proteins, fats (oils) and carbohydrates. According to the Food and Nutrition Board of the National Academy of Sciences, at least 50 to 100 grams (200 to 400 calories) of digestible carbohydrates per day are desirable to offset undesirable metabolic responses. Although this board made no distinction between *refined* and *unrefined* carbohydrates, a number of research studies, including those by Cheraskin and Ringsdorf,[1] show that unrefined carbohydrates (vegetables, fruits and whole grains) promote health. By contrast, their studies indicate that refined carbohydrates (cane, beet and corn sugars and syrups, and white flour) promote disease, including dental caries, high blood pressure, emotional disorders and susceptibility to infection.

I met Cheraskin over 10 years ago at a medical meeting in Miami and became one of his fans. I began following the Cheraskin-Ringsdorf recommendations in prescribing diets for my patients. And I urged them to eat more vegetables, fruits and whole grains along with a variety of other wholesome foods, including nuts and seeds, some dairy products, eggs and meats, especially chicken and fish.

About the same time, I began to notice that *children who consumed diets loaded with sugar and corn syrup became irritable, nervous and hyperactive.* And when these foods were removed from their diets, their symptoms would improve. Also, many of my adult patients would comment,

> "When I cut down on my sweets and other junk food, I feel better . . . less nervousness, irritability and fatigue."

At the same meeting where I met Cheraskin, I had dinner with Nathan Pritikin, the Californian who reported that diets containing

80% complex carbohydrates (400 or more grams of complex carbohydrate per day) would help people with all sorts of health disorders. Included among these were high blood pressure, hardening of the arteries and adult onset diabetes.

A couple of years later, Pritikin asked me to serve as a member of the Advisory Board of the Pritikin Research Foundation. I visited the Pritikin center in California twice and was impressed with the "fantastic" results obtained by many people I met who had followed the Pritikin program.

Soon thereafter, my good friend, Jacksonian H. A. ("Rich") Richardson who had suffered from the severe and persistent chest pain called "angina", learned of the Pritikin program. One of his sons commented,

> "Dad had to take nitroglycerin every day. His pain bothered him even at rest and during the night. He had to sit up in bed. He couldn't sleep."

Complete heart studies, including catheterization at the Ochsner Clinic in New Orleans, showed complete blockage of one of Rich's major arteries and 60 to 90 percent blockage of the others. Open heart surgery was initially recommended (in 1975). Yet the severity of Rich's heart disease was such that he was subsequently told,

> "You'd be a poor operative risk."

So Rich kept taking his nitroglycerin and his pain continued. About a year later, Rich and his wife, Rosemary, read a report in an Atlanta paper about the Pritikin program. They went to California, spent a month eating the high carbohydrate diet and started walking. Today, 7 years later, 70-year-old Rich walks three to six miles a day and works almost 12 hours a day, six days a week, running a highly successful business. He takes no medicine and experiences no pain unless he walks too fast up a hill. One of his sons commented,

> "Every person who works for dad has to push to keep up with him!"

Soon afterward, an across-the-street neighbor, Turner Bridges (then age 69), was told by his physician,

> "You have diabetes. And your cholesterol is too high . . . over 250."

On a modified Pritikin diet, Turner's diabetes has vanished and his cholesterol has fallen to 165. Turner travels, plays golf regularly (no golf cart) and enjoys better health than many men half his age.

For over 10 years, I've admired Roger Williams, Ph.D. of the University of Texas in Austin, Ross Hume Hall, Ph.D. of McMasters University in Hamilton, Ontario, and author Beatrice Trum Hunter of Hillsboro, New Hampshire. These professionals have stressed the importance of nutritious, wholesome, truly natural foods, including vegetables, fruits and whole grains. And I've read their books from cover to cover several times.

Each of these professionals say in effect,

> "Avoid fabricated and processed foods of all sorts, especially those containing sugar, processed fat, food coloring and other additives."

Moreover, I've been impressed by the growing interest of both professionals and non-professionals in diets containing less meat, eggs and fat-laden dairy products, and featuring more vegetables, fruits and grains. For example, Jane Brody, award-winning science writer and personal health columnist of *The New York Times*, and author of *Jane Brody's Nutrition Book*[12], commented,

> "Even if you have no interest in vegetarianism, *there's no reason why you should have animal protein at every meal or even every day.*"

So with this sort of background, I had to re-orient my thinking and make a 180° turn-around before I could recommend diets *high in protein and fat* and *low in carbohydrate*. Yet, beginning in 1979 when I saw a number of my patients improve on such diets, I became convinced of their value in my patients with yeast-connected illnesses.

My initial diet for most patients contained 100 grams of carbohydrate. If the patient improved rapidly, I increased the carbohydrate content to 150 grams . . . ocassionally more. I recommend more vegetables, whole grains and fruits, rather than foods containing sugar or white flour products.

If the patient wasn't improving, I would occasionally suggest a diet with a carbohydrate content of only 60 to 80 grams. After a week or two, if things were better, I recommended additional "good" carbohydrates. In dealing with children, I limited only the foods containing sugar, corn syrup and white flour. I allowed any vegetable, fruit or whole grain product, unless the child showed an allergic reaction to a permitted food.

Helping my candida patients with their diets hasn't been easy for me . . . or for them. And in talking to one of them recently, I commented,

"The more I learn about the relationship of diet to human illness, the more excited I become. Yet, sometimes it seems the more I know, the more unanswered questions I have."

In my experience, foods which cause problems are those which contain yeasts, molds or refined carbohydrate products, especially sugar. And I've found that many of my patients tolerate "good" carbohydrates found in vegetables, whole grains and fruits, unless they're allergic to these foods. Yet, I was surprised to find that other of my patients did not improve until and unless they restricted all carbohydrates. Then, after a few weeks, as they improved, most found they could experiment and add more carbohydrates without developing symptoms.

Here are other reports of the efficacy of low carbohydrate diets. A physician who developed a great interest in yeast-connected illness because of his own severe health problems commented,

"As I've struggled to overcome candida and regain my health, I've learned that I must keep the total carbohydrate content of my diet at a low level. To accomplish this, I greatly restrict my intake of fruits and grains."

Moreover, several of my own patients have recently reported,

"When I eat too many carbohydrates, even the 'good ones', my symptoms flare." One patient, Lynn, who suffered with severe fatigue, bloating, abdominal stress and other candida-connected health problems, had this to say, "If I eat fruits or grains, I develop immediate symptoms."

Here's still more: In March, 1983, I met Betty Flora who commented,

"Stopping all gluten-containing foods (wheat, rye, barley and oats) and all fruits was an important factor in helping me conquer my yeast-connected health problems.

"Let's go back to the glutenous grains and consider their relationship to candida. I suspect that yeast needs two things . . . something to nest in and something to feed on . . . gluten is what they love to nest in. Then consider that, nearly always, grains are flavored with something sweet. The sugar, honey, syrup and molasses serve as food for the yeast.

"Another simple view is to picture how we start yeast bread. We put gluten flour and yeast together, but we have to add sugar for the yeast to feed on, then look out for the doubling and redoubling in bulk. It's just the same in my body. If I put any of the glutenous products into my body, along with the usual honey or molasses, plus sweetening in my heavenly home-made bran muffins . . . I seem to furnish yeast within my body what it needs . . . and my weight gain is astronomical."

Betty also told me of the observations of Shirley Lorenzani, Ph.D. of St. Petersburg, Florida,

"I'm exhilarated over the help patients are obtaining when they follow a treatment program designed to overcome candida. Although many of our patients improve when they go on a yeast-free diet and stop eating junk food, others must limit their intake of many carbohydrates.

"We have found that most patients with yeast-connected illness improve more rapidly if they eat only vegetables, eggs, meat, poultry, seafood, butter, oil, and small servings of rice and millet for the first eight weeks of their program. We've also found the cytotoxic food test useful in helping our patients identify and avoid foods which may be causing adverse reactions." (see also pages 119-120)

Another point of view: In discussing the diets he recommends for patients with yeast-related illness, Dr. Elmer Cranton of Troutdale, Virginia said,

"Many patients are sensitive to common foods they eat every day, including not only whole grains and citrus, but also milk and egg. Accordingly, in my practice, I begin by using Diet A in your book, *Tracking Down Hidden Food Allergy*"[13].

(See, also pages 127-130.)

Perhaps in prescribing diets for candida-related illness, we may resemble the 18th century British physician, James Lind. Dr. Lind found that he could prevent and treat the dreaded (and often fatal) disease scurvy by providing sailors with a regular supply of limes and/or other fresh fruits and vegetables. But, it wasn't until 1929 . . . almost 200 years later, following the discovery of vitamin C by Hungarian biochemist, Albert Szent Györgi . . . that medical science learned why limes worked.

Those of us treating candida-related illness today face a similar situation; *we know that dietary changes help the patient with candida, but we do not understand all the mechanisms involved.*

On the pages that follow, you'll find instructions for making changes in your diet which will help you conquer your candida-

71

related health problems. And I'd like to emphasize the following points:

1. Each person is unique and your dietary requirements may differ in many ways from the requirements of others with yeast-connected health problems.
2. Your diet should contain liberal amounts of nutritious foods from a wide variety of sources.
3. You should avoid foods such as breads, to which yeast has been added, and foods which contain molds or yeasts such as vinegar and all cheeses. You should also avoid yeast-containing beverages, especially wine and beer, and yeast-containing vitamin preparations.
4. You should also avoid margarine and "junk foods" . . . foods which are refined, overly-processed and loaded with sugar, salt, food coloring, additives and hardened (hydrogenated or partially hydrogenated) vegetable oil.

In preparing these diet instructions, I emphasize the foods you *can eat*, along with admonitions about the foods you should avoid.

The first and easiest of the diets I use in my practice is the **Candida Control Diet**. This diet emphasizes foods from a wide variety of sources and *restricts only those foods which contain yeast, honey, cane sugar, beet sugar, corn sugar, fructose and other refined carbohydrates*. It does not limit your intake of the good carbohydrate foods . . . fresh vegetables and fruits, freshly squeezed juices and whole grains.

If you follow the **Candida Control Diet** and do not improve, it may be because you're troubled by adverse reactions to foods you're eating every day. Or the yeasts in your digestive tract may be thriving on carbohydrates, including those which I've termed, "good carbohydrate" (high carbohydrate vegetables, grains and fruits).

The second diet I use and recommend is the **Low Carbohydrate Diet**. This diet is preferred by many physicians and I recommend it as an initial diet for adults with long-standing and severe yeast-connected health problems. This diet avoids sugar, corn syrup, fructose, honey, fruits, milk and foods containing yeasts and molds and limits your daily intake of whole grains, and vegetables with high carbohydrate content, including potatoes, yams and corn. You'll find instructions for carrying out such a diet in the section entitled, **Low Carbohydrate Diet**.

A third diet is described under the heading, **Fruit-free, Sugar-Free, Yeast-Free Diet** (pages 117-118.) (Research studies by John W. Rippon, Ph. D., of the University of Chicago indicate that fruits encourage yeast growth.)

A fourth even more restrictive diet is the **Sugar-Free, Yeast-Free, Fruit-Free, Grain-Free, Nut-Free, Milk-Free Diet** (see pages 119-120) recommended by the Price-Pottenger Nutrition Foundation (PPNF) of California. Although I've had little experience with this diet, some professionals feel it is essential in controlling candida in their patients, especially those who haven't improved on other treatment regimens. (see also pages 70-71)

As you review these comments and especially after you read and study the instructions, I'm sure you'll have a lot of questions. Here are some of them:

"How strictly do I need to adhere to the diet?"

"Do I start on the **Candida Control Diet** or would I get better quicker if I started on the **Low Carbohydrate Diet.**†Or should I do the **Fruit-Free, Sugar-Free, Yeast-Free Diet**, or that even more difficult diet which allows only vegetables, meat, fish, eggs and butter?"

"How will I manage eating out?"

"What am I going to drink besides water? Will a cup of coffee really hurt me?"

"How about health food teas?" (See also page 94)

"How about an occasional glass of wine or beer?"

"How about breads? Where will I get them since all grocery store breads contain yeast?"

"How about the diet drinks? Are they safe?"

"How about those left-overs? Can't I ever use them? Does mold always grow in them?" (See also page 94.)

"Will 'just a little sugar' hurt? And what about the sugar substitutes like saccharin and Equal®? Are they safe? (See especially pages 294, 295.)

Some of these questions can easily be answered. Yet others can't. But because all of these subjects are important, I discuss them further on pages 87-95, 117-125, 277-298.

---

† Rebecca Davis, R.D., a nutritionist who has worked with me for many years, commented: "Vegetables, fruits and whole grains (complex carbohydrates) provide many essential nutrients. And diets high in complex carbohydrates are consumed by many healthy people. I feel that any diet which restricts such carbohydrates should be supervised by a qualified professional and shouldn't be continued for long periods of time."

11

The Candida Control Diet

Foods You Can Eat

Vegetables

Asparagus
Beets
Broccoli
Brussel sprouts
Cabbage
Carrots
Cauliflower
Celery
Cucumbers
Eggplant
Green peppers

Lettuce
Onions
Parsley
Peas, beans & legumes
Tomatoes, fresh
Summer & winter squash
Zucchini, acorn, & butternut squash
White potatoes
Sweet potatoes
Radishes
Okra
Parsnip
Corn

All Fresh Vegetables

Greens:
  Turnip
  Spinach
  Mustard
  Beet
  Collards
  Kale

Fruits (fresh)†

Apple
Avocado
Banana
Grapes
Peach
Pear
Pineapple
Apricot

Berries (all kinds)
Cherries
Grapefruit
Mango
Nectarine
Orange
Papaya
Plum

All Fresh Fruits

---

† Studies by John W. Rippon, Ph.D., indicate that in spite of their fiber content, carbohydrates in fruits are broken down to simple sugars more readily than carbohydrates in vegetables. Accordingly, fruits may promote the growth of candida in your digestive tract. (see pages vii, viii, 42, 73, 117-120 for a further discussion.)

Foods You Can Eat †

Meats

Beef	Squirrel
Pork	Rabbit
Chicken	Quail
Turkey	Duck
Lamb	Goose
Veal	Cornish hen
Egg	Pheasant
Tuna	and other game birds

Salmon
and other fresh fish
Clam
Lobster
Shrimp
Crab
Oysters

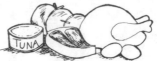

Meats and Eggs
(any but bacon, sausage, ham, hot dogs or luncheon meats)

Beverages
Milk‡
Water

Beverages (milk and water)

Whole Grains
Barley
Corn
Millet
Oats
Rice
Wheat

Cereal Grains, Bread and Muffins (containing no yeast, honey or sugar)

Nuts, Seeds & Oils
(**unprocessed**)
Almonds
Brazil nuts
Cashews
Filberts
Pecans
Pumpkin seeds
Oils (cold pressed)
   Almond
   Apricot
   Avocado
   Corn
   Linseed
   Olive
   Safflower
   Sesame
   Sunflower
Butter

Unprocessed Nuts, Seeds and Oils

---

† See Shopping Tips, page 85, Food Sources, page 86, Recipes, pages 111-116, and "Other Comments About the CANDIDA-CONTROL Diet," pages 87-93.

‡ Because of its high content of the simple carbohydrate lactose, milk also promotes yeast growth. For further comments on milk see pages 100, 293-294.

Foods You Must Avoid

Sugar & Sugar-containing Foods: Sugar & other quick-acting carbohydrates, including sucrose, fructose, maltose, lactose, glycogen, glucose, mannitol, sorbitol, galactose, monosaccharides and polysaccharides. Also avoid honey, molasses, maple syrup, maple sugar, date sugar and turbinado sugar.

Yeast, Breads & Pastries: Raised baked goods, including breads, rolls, coffee cakes and pastries containing baker's yeast.

Alcoholic Beverages: Wine, beer, whiskey, brandy, gin, rum, vodka and other fermented liquors and liqueurs. Also, fermented beverages such as cider and root beer.

Malt Products: Malted milk drinks, cereals and candy. (Malt is sprouted grain that is kiln-dried and used in the preparation of many processed foods and beverages.)

Condiments, Sauces and Vinegar-containing foods: Mustard, ketchup, Worcestershire®, Accent® (monosodium glutamate); steak, barbecue, chili, shrimp and soy sauces; pickles, picked vegetables, relishes, green olives, sauerkraut, horseradish, mince meat and tamari. Also avoid sprouts. Vinegar of all kinds and vinegar-containing foods such as mayonnaise and salad dressing. (Freshly squeezed lemon juice may be used as a substitute for vinegar in salad dressings prepared with unprocessed vegetable oil.)

Processed & Smoked Meats: Pickled and smoked meats and fish including sausages, hot dogs, corned beef, pastrami and pickled tongue.

Dried & Candied Fruits: Raisins, apricots, dates, prunes, figs, pineapple.

Left-overs: Molds grow in left-over food unless it's properly refrigerated. Freezing is better.

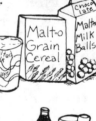

Foods You Must Avoid

Fruit Juices: Either canned, bottled or frozen, including orange juice, grape juice, apple juice, tomato juice, pineapple juice. (Exception: freshly prepared juice.)

Coffee and Tea: Regular coffee, instant coffee and teas of all sorts, including herb teas.

Melons: Watermelon, honeydew melon and especially cantaloupe.†

Edible Fungi: All types of mushrooms, morels and truffles.

Cheeses: All cheeses, including Swiss cheese, cottage cheese and cream cheese. (Moldy cheeses such as Roquefort are the worst.) Prepared foods, including Velveeta®, macaroni and cheese, Cheezits® and other cheese-containing snacks. Also buttermilk, sour cream and sour milk products.††

Yeasts: Brewer's yeast, baker's yeast and all foods whose preparation obviously depend on yeast.

Vitamins & Minerals: B-complex vitamins, selenium products (unless labeled "yeast-free" and "sugar-free").

Antibiotics:††† Specifically, antibacterial antibiotics, including penicillin, streptomycin, ampicillin, amoxicillin, Keflex®, Ceclor®, Septra® and Bactrim®.

Packaged and Processed Foods: Canned, bottled, boxed and other packaged and processed foods usually contain yeast or refined sugar products. Also avoid enriched flour products.

Nuts: Peanuts and peanut products usually contain mold. So do pistachios.

---

† Porous skin of cantaloupe is especially apt to be contaminated with mold. However, careful washing before cutting may enable melons to be tolerated.
†† Many individuals tolerate fruit-free, sugar-free, yogurt. For a full discussion of yogurt and it's role in controlling candida see page 266.
††† Antibiotics are indicated in treating certain infections. However, most infections are caused by viruses and do not respond to antibiotic therapy.

Candida Control Diet
Meal Suggestions
BREAKFAST

Ground beef patty
Scrambled eggs
Grits with butter
Applesauce muffin†

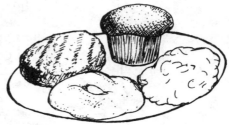

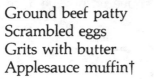

Pork chop
Sliced potatoes
Whole wheat biscuit†
Grapefruit

Toasted rice cakes with
butter
Sliced banana
Cashew nuts

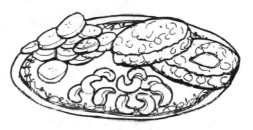

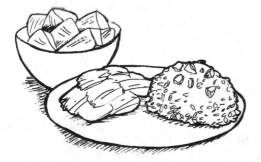

Brown rice with butter
and chopped almonds
Tuna, water pack
Fresh pineapple

---

† See Recipes, pages 111-116.

Candida Control Diet

Meal Suggestions

BREAKFAST

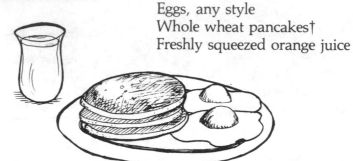

Eggs, any style
Whole wheat pancakes†
Freshly squeezed orange juice

Barley cereal with
banana and pecans
Milk
Fish (baked or broiled)

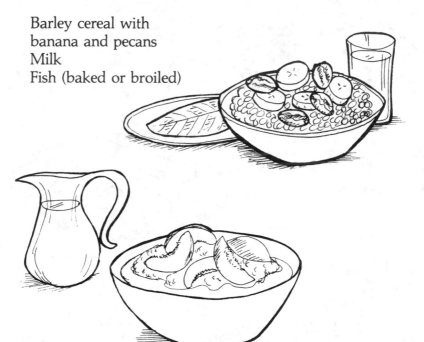

Hot oatmeal with peaches (fresh or frozen,
without sugar), and cashews
Milk

---

† See Recipes, pages 111-116.

Candida Control Diet
Meal Suggestions

LUNCH

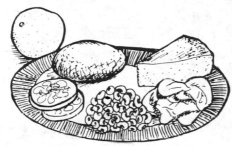

Salmon patty
Cornbread†
Boiled Cabbage
Blackeyed peas
Sliced tomatoes
Orange

Fish Cakes
Steamed cauliflower
Boiled okra
Oat cakes†
Strawberries

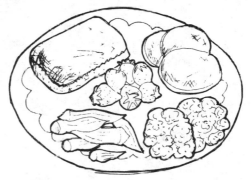

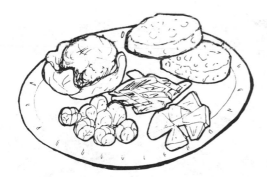

Tuna salad on lettuce
Rice cakes†
Steamed green beans
Boiled Brussel sprouts
Fresh pineapple

† See Recipes, pages 111-116.

Candida Control Diet

Meal Suggestions

LUNCH

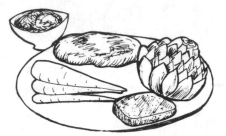

Swiss steak
Steamed artichoke
Turnip greens
Raw carrots
Corn bread†

Chicken salad†
Rice soup†
Spinach
Rice biscuits
Apple

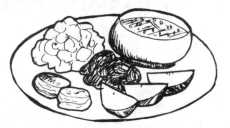

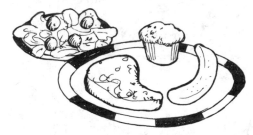

Pork chop
Lettuce & tomato salad
Applesauce muffin
Baked banana

Meat loaf
Barley soup†
Celery and carrots
Whole wheat biscuits
Pear

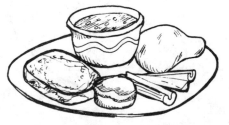

---

† See Recipes, pages 111-116.

Candida Control Diet

Meal Suggestions

MAIN MEAL

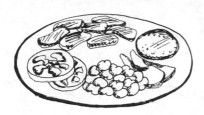

Sauteed liver†
Lima beans
Baked acorn squash†
Sliced tomato
Banana oat cake†

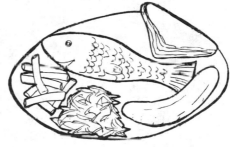

Broiled fish
Cabbage & carrot slaw†
Wax beans
Whole wheat popovers†
Baked banana

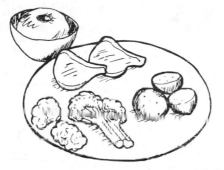

Broiled lamb chops
Steamed cauliflower
Steamed broccoli
Boiled potatoes
Baked apple

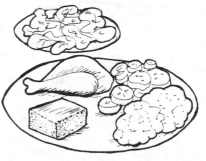

Rock cornish hen
Steamed carrots and peas
Wild rice
Corn bread†
Papaya

---

† See Recipes, pages 111-116.

Candida Control Diet
Meal Suggestions
MAIN MEAL

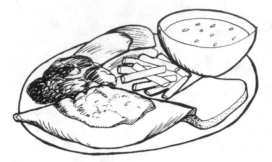

Roast duck
Spinach
Barley soup†
Sweet potato
Steamed green beans
Corn bread†

Broiled steak
Baked potato
Lettuce, tomato, cucumber salad
   with freshly squeezed lemon
   juice & safflower or linseed oil
   dressing
Lima beans
Spoon bread†
Fresh strawberries

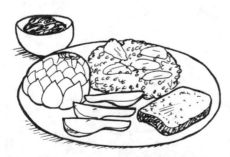

Easy chicken and rice†
Steamed artichoke
Turnip greens
Corn bread†
Pear

† See Recipes, pages 111-116.

Shopping Tips

1. Feature whole foods.

2. Avoid foods labeled "enriched" (they contain yeast).

3. Since many, and perhaps most canned, packaged and processed foods contain hidden ingredients, including sugar, dextrose and other carbohydrate products, avoid them.

4. If you must use canned or packaged foods, **Read Labels Carefully**.

5. Avoid processed, smoked or cured meats, such as salami, wieners, bacon, sausage, hotdogs, etc., since they often contain sugar, spices, yeast and other additives.

6. Use fresh fruits and vegetables. Commercially canned products often contain yeasts and added sugar.†

7. Avoid bottled, frozen and canned juices. If you wish juice, buy fresh fruit and prepare your own juice.†

8. Most commercially available nuts are roasted in vegetable oil and contain additives. Buy nuts in the shell, or shelled nuts from a natural food store. Avoid peanuts since they contain mold. (And nuts of all kinds, like other foods, may become contaminated with molds.)

9. All commercial breads, cakes and crackers contain yeast. If you wish yeast-free breads, you'll have to obtain them from a special bakery or bake your own.†† Arden, Chico San or Golden Harvest Rice Cakes contain no sugar or yeast. Most children and adults like them. They're good with nut butters. Also San-Esu Rice Snacks (plain or sesame) and Kame Rice Crackers. (Usually found at natural food stores.)

10. Use cold pressed vegetable oils (such as sunflower, safflower, linseed and corn). (To make salad dressing, combine the oil with fresh lemon juice.)

11. Buy whole grains (barley, corn, millet, oats, rice and wheat) from a natural food store. Grains can be an important ingredient of a nutritious breakfast. Barley, rice and other grains can also be used in various ways at other meals. Barley or rice casseroles are especially tasty.††

---

† For a further discussion of fruits and juice, see pages 88-89, 93, 117-120.
†† See Recipes, pages 111-116.

Food sources

Rice cakes
Arden Organic
99 Pond Road
Asheville, N.C. 28806

Vegetable oils, wheat, oats, rye
Arrowhead Mills, Inc.
Hereford, Texas 79045

Rice crackers (contain whole brown rice, sesame seeds & salt)
Chico San, Inc.
1144 West First Street
Chico, Calif. 95926

Puffed corn, rice, wheat, and millet
El Molino Mills
City of Industry, Calif. 91746

Ener-G Rice Mix®, Ener-G Egg Replacer®, Jolly Joan Soyquik®
Ener-G Foods, Inc.
P.O. Box 24723
Seattle, Washington 98124

Vegetable oils, cashew butter, almond butter
Hain Pure Food
Company, Inc.
Los Angeles, Calif. 90061

Potato chips (contain potato, safflower oil & salt. No additives)
Health Valley Natural
Foods, Inc.
700 Union
Montebello, Calif. 90640

Bottled water, vegetables, nuts, whole grains, flours
Shiloh Farms
Sulphur Springs, Ark. 72768

Unprocessed nuts
Tropical Nut & Fruit Co.
11517-A Cordage Rd.
P.O. Box 7507
Charlotte, N.C. 28217

Also check with your local natural food store. They may be able to supply these and other yeast free, sugar free foods.

Additional Helpful Suggestions

Many individuals with yeast-connected health problems improve . . . often dramatically . . . when they avoid the major yeast-containing foods including raised breads, cheeses, mushrooms and dried fruits. They improve even more when they avoid alcoholic beverages, including wine and beer, and stop eating foods containing significant amounts of cane sugar, beet sugar, corn syrup, fructose, dextrose or honey. Moreover, such individuals can consume limited quantities of foods and beverages which contain a small amount of yeast, molds or sugar.

For example, such persons may eat a low-sugar dry cereal such as Cheerios® without developing symptoms because of the sugar or malt. And they may tolerate a morning cup of coffee or afternoon pot of tea, even though the berries or leaves of these beverages contain mold.

Others with candida-related illness (especially those with severe disorders) pay for any dietary infraction. And they may not achieve maximum improvement until they avoid all mold-containing foods. So they must stay away from coffee, teas, spices, sprouts, condiments and unfrozen left-over foods (mold quickly grows on any food which isn't eaten as soon as it's prepared). They must also avoid any and every food which contains sugar or yeast *in any form.*

Still others must carry out food allergy detective work. They must identify and avoid (or otherwise treat) all foods that cause adverse or allergic reactions. Common offenders include milk, egg, wheat, corn and soy. However, any food can be a trouble-maker, including beef, pork, lettuce, chicken, apple, tomato, banana, grape and other foods.

When an adverse reaction is caused by a food such as lobster, shrimp or cashew nuts, it can usually be identified with ease. However, when such reactions are caused by foods that are eaten frequently, the relationship of the food to a person's symptoms is rarely suspected.

To identify hidden food allergies requires a carefully designed and appropriately executed elimination diet, as described in my book, *Tracking Down Hidden Food Allergy*[13]. (See, also pages 127-130.)

Each person differs from every other person. **YOU ARE UNIQUE.** In following the anti-candida diet, *use a trial and error approach.*

Most of my patients with candida-related illness, as they improve, can follow a less rigid diet, especially if they're following other measures to regain their health. Included are the use of nutritional supplements and exercise, and avoiding exposure to environmental chemicals and mold spores. (See pages 55-64 and 131-155 for a further discussion of these factors.)

Why do sweetened foods and beverages cause symptoms?:
During the past 20 years, I've heard countless patients say,

> "When I eat sweets, I feel spaced out, irritable, jittery or depressed."

And many a parent has commented,

> "When Johnny eats sugar, he becomes hyperactive and unable to concentrate."

Why do such reactions occur? What is the mechanism? Here are a few possibilities:

1. When you eat refined sugars, you may be feeding yeast germs in your digestive tract and causing them to multiply. As a result toxins are produced which may cause symptoms all over the body.

2. Diets containing large amounts of refined sugar cause your pancreas to put out extra insulin. As a result, rapid up and down fluctuations occur in your blood and brain sugar levels producing nervousness, weakness, irritability, drowsiness and other symptoms of hypoglycemia.

3. If you fill up on sugar-laden foods, chances are you won't consume enough essential nutrients, including calcium and magnesium. Your diet may also be deficient in other essential vitamins and trace minerals, including vitamin B-1, vitamin B-6, chromium, zinc, essential amino acids, essential fatty acids and other nutrients. Such nutrients participate in various body enzyme systems and serve as precursors in the manufacture of hormones and neurotransmitters (chemicals your brain requires to function properly).

4. You may be allergic to sucrose and other sugars derived from a particular botanical source (cane, beet, corn or maple). In my own practice, dozens of my patients have commented, "Cane sugar products cause reactions, yet I can take beet or corn

sugar." Or, "Foods sweetened with corn syrup make me irritable and nervous, yet other sweetened foods don't bother me." Other clinical ecologists have made similar observations. (For a further discussion of adverse reactions to different sugars, see page 200.)

Yeast and mold-containing foods: *Avoiding yeasts and molds in your diet isn't easy.* Molds are everywhere . . . indoors and outdoors. Although dampness and darkness promote mold growth, as do basements and cellars, *molds can grow on any food, including fruits, vegetables, nuts, meats, spices and left-overs.* Although heating . . . even boiling or processing . . . may kill live molds, mold products may be left behind which may cause problems for some individuals with candida-related health problems.

Accordingly, in following the candida-control diet, you'll need to avoid the foods with high mold and yeast content until your immune system recovers and most of your health problems disappear. Then you can experiment and try a less rigid diet.

Here are further comments on foods that usually contain yeasts and molds: (See also page 94 for an additional discussion of yeast and mold-containing foods.)

Fruit juices: Most fruit juices, including frozen, bottled or canned, are prepared from fruits that have been allowed to stand in bins, barrels and other containers for periods ranging from an hour on up to several days or weeks. Although juice processors discard fruits that are obviously spoiled by mold, most fruits used for juice making contain mold. Even freshly pre- 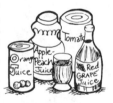 pared juices or whole fresh fruit may promote yeast growth accor ding to yeast and mold expert John W. Rippon, Ph.D. (see pages 117-119.)

Coffee & tea: These popular beverages, including the health food teas, are prepared from plant products. Such products are subject to mold contamination. How much is uncertain. If you feel you can't get along without your coffee or tea, you'll have to experiment and see what happens. Some herbal teas have been reported to have therapeutic value. A California physician who has been using Taheebo® tea in treating some of her patients commented,

"I've found that Taheebo® tea helps. I've been using it since November, 1982. It seems to help, especially, in clearing nasal symptoms."

89

Alcoholic beverages: Wines, beers and other alcoholic beverages contain high levels of yeast contamination so must be avoided.

One physician consultant who has studied candida-related illness extensively commented,

> "I feel people who crave alcohol probably suffer from candida-related illness. And an alcoholic almost certainly has the candida problem."

Other beverages:

> "What's a person to drink?"

asked one of my patients.

> "You've taken away my beer, my Scotch, my coffee, my tea, my cokes and my juices. That leaves only water. Isn't there something else? How about diet drinks?"

Diet drinks have no nutritional value. Moreover, they often contain caffeine, food coloring, phosphates, saccharin and other ingredients which disagree with many individuals. However, since these beverages do not contain mold, individuals with candida-related problems may tolerate them. If you use them, don't go overboard.

Many people with chronic health problems, especially those with chemical sensitivity, require bottled or distilled water to remain symptom-free. Others find they can tolerate tap water if they install a water filter in their home.

In an article in the Summer, 1982 issue of *The Long Island Pediatrician* (published by Chapter 2, District II, American Academy of Pediatrics) entitled, "How Safe is Long Island Drinking Water," Frances S. Sterrett,[14] Ph.D., Professor of Chemistry, Hofstra University, commented,

> "Several hundred different organic chemical substances have been found in a variety of drinking waters. For this reason, I and many other people on Long Island and in many parts of the country filter our drinking water through an activated carbon water filter . . . Water consumed by infants and small children should be filtered through activated carbon and boiled because cumulative effects of low level contaminants are more critical at such an early age."

(Information on water filters can be found in the book, *Water Fit to*

Drink, by Carol Keough, Rodale Press, Inc., Emmaus, Pa., 1980, and in the February, 1983 issue of *Consumer Reports*).

Left-overs: Such foods provide a rich breeding ground for yeasts and molds. Molds are one of the major micro-organisms causing foods to spoil, and all foods spoil. Although refrigeration retards mold growth, even refrigerated foods develop mold contamination. So prepare only as much food as you need and eat it promptly, or freeze left-overs.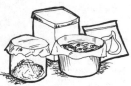

At the July, 1982 Dallas Candida Conference, Dr. Francis Waickman of Cuyahoga Falls, Ohio commented,

> "Several of my mold sensitive patients must eat foods immediately after they're cooked. Left-overs always cause their symptoms to flare."

Whether or not you can eat left-overs will depend on the severity of your health problems and how sensitive you are to mold. Some individuals can eat left-overs without developing symptoms, while others cannot. It takes trial and error experimenting to find out which foods cause trouble and which ones do not.

Spices & condiments: These dietary ingredients are usually loaded with mold and should be avoided or approached with caution. 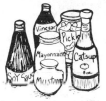 Limited quantities of salt and juice from a freshly squeezed lemon are your safest food flavoring agents. And freshly squeezed lemon juice, plus unprocessed vegetable oil, makes a healthy, nutritious salad dressing. Moreover, unprocessed vegetable oils, especially flaxseed or linseed oil, safflower or sunflower oil, are rich in essential fatty acids which are important precursors of substances your body requires for proper functioning. (For further discussion of fatty acids, see pages 137-138, 246.)

Cereal grains: Cereal grains, including oats, wheat, rice, barley, corn and millet, especially those found in natural food stores, are excellent sources of vitamins and minerals. Moreover, such unprocessed grains contain no sugar. However, like other foods, some mold contamination may occur. Nevertheless, such grains can play an important role in meeting your nutritional needs. (For additional comments on grains, see pages 69,137.)

How about dry cereals? These cereal grains . . . even the best of them . . . have been processed and subjected to high heat. Accordingly, they're much less desirable than hot cereals you prepare at home made from whole grain. Moreover, most dry cereals are loaded with sugar, malt and food coloring.

Several years ago, on the "Today Show", Dr. Art Ulene showed a box of one of the popular cereals advertised for children and said,

> "This 14 ounce box contains 80 teaspoons of sugar. In fact, sugar is the main ingredient. And some two dozen of these cereals contain over 40% sugar."

If, in spite of their limited nutritional value, you decide on a dry cereal, get sugar-free Shredded Wheat®. Cereals which contain less than 6% added sugar include Cheerios®, Puffed Rice®, Wheat Chex®, Puffed Wheat®, Post Toasties®, Product 19®, and Special K®. However, I don't recommend them for anticandida diets as many contain malt and added yeast-derived B vitamins.

Breads: Nearly all commercially-available breads, cakes, crackers and cookies contain yeast or sugar and cause symptoms in patients with candida-related problems. So they should be avoided. However, a few yeast-free and sugar-free products may be found in natural food stores and specialty departments of some supermarkets.†

Nuts: Nuts are loaded with good nutrients, especially trace minerals. However, most commercially available nuts on supermarket shelves contain additives of various sorts, including dextrose (corn sugar). So use unprocessed nuts. Ideally, nuts should be freshly shelled, since nuts stored for long periods of time (like fruits and other foods) attract mold growth. Avoid peanuts and peanut products since they're contaminated with mold.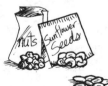

Candies & sweets: Many people crave sugar, especially people with the candida problem. In fact, New York pediatrician, allergist and clinical ecologist, Morton Teich commented,

> "Sugar craving is one of the leading symptoms that leads me to suspect candida-related illness in my patients."

† See pages 111-117 for recipes and suggestions for yeast-free and sugar-free baked products.

What to do about it? Stay away from sugar-containing foods. After your immune system and your health improve, you may be able to cheat occasionally. An alternate: Use bananas and other fruits to prepare cookies, cakes and other sweetened foods. If you'd like a guide to help you prepare such foods, get a copy of the "all-natural, fruit-sweetened cookbook" by Karen E. Barkie entitled *Sweet & Sugar Free*, St. Martin's Press, 175 Fifth Ave., New York, New York 10010, 1982.

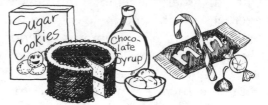

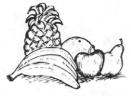

Fresh fruits & vegetables, including salads: Since molds grow everywhere, including the outer surfaces of lettuce, tomatoes and other fruits and vegetables, such foods may cause reactions in highly susceptible individuals. To lessen mold contamination, a Massachusetts physician suggests cleaning foods with a weak Clorox® solution. (See page 256.) And he said,

"Although the fumes from Clorox® bother many chemically-sensitive patients, a person can avoid such reactions by using a nose clip while preparing the solution."

Eating out: If you're like most people, you live "on the run" and eat foods away from home. What's the answer? Do the best you can. And during the early weeks and months of your candida-control program, you may need to do a lot of brown-bagging (see pages 121-122). And when you eat out, you'll need to make your selections carefully, so as to avoid foods that trigger your symptoms.

In my own practice, I've found that most patients improve when they avoid sugar, junk food, yeast-containing vitamins and the major mold-containing foods. Yet, some patients, especially during the early phases of their treatment program, *must avoid all foods which contain yeasts, molds or sugars and restrict their intake of all carbohydrates.* Still others with severe yeast-connected illness have found they must avoid all gluten-containing grains and avoid or sharply limit their intake of fruits. (See, also, page 119.)

More on Yeast and Mold-containing Foods

Many (and perhaps most) of my patients with yeast-connected health disorders develop symptoms when they consume foods or beverages which contain yeasts and molds. Wine and moldy cheeses seem to be especially common offenders.

Yet, during the past year, a number of my patients have reported they tolerated cheeses, teas, peanuts, mushrooms and other yeast-containing foods. However, other dietary cheating (like eating a sugar-rich food) would invariably produce fatigue, bloating, headache, vaginitis, irritability or other symptoms.

I reported these observations to mold authority John W. Rippon, Ph.D. who commented

> "Eating a yeast-containing food doesn't make candida organisms grow and multiply. So when your patients develop symptoms from yeasty foods, they do so because they're allergic to yeast products." (See page 118.)

Accordingly, as you improve and want to "try your wings" and cheat on your diet (if *you aren't bothered by mold allergies*), consuming yeast or mold-containing food or beverages would seem to be a good place to start. But do it cautiously and don't go overboard!

12

The Low Carbohydrate Diet[†]

Foods You Can Eat Freely

. . . Meats & eggs

Unprocessed meats contain insignificant amounts of carbohydrate. Do not use luncheon meats or breaded meats. For a lower cholesterol intake, choose poultry and fish.

Chicken
Turkey
Salmon
Tuna
Any fresh or frozen fish that is not breaded
Beef, all lean cuts
Veal
Pork, all lean cuts
Lamb
Eggs

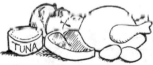

---

† *Complex carbohydrates, including vegetables, whole grains and fruits, are nutritious, health-promoting foods for most people.* Yet, if you're bothered by a yeast-connected health disorder, you'll need to restrict your intake of carbohydrates until you improve. *You should especially avoid sugar, corn syrup, fruits and milk* (milk contains lactose, a carbohydrate which encourages candida growth).

Although the carbohydrate content of fruits and milk are listed in this section along with the carbohydrate content of other foods, the MEAL SUGGESTIONS and the 7-DAY MEAL PLAN contain no fruits or milk. After a few weeks, when your immune system improves and your candida is brought under control, you can try rotating fruits and milk into your diet and see if you tolerate them.

Foods You Can Eat Freely

. . . Low carbohydrate vegetables
Most of these vegetables contain relatively little carbohydrate. They can be fresh or frozen, and you can eat them cooked or raw.

	Portion	Grams of Carbohydrate
Asparagus	1 cup	5
Beets	1 cup	12
Broccoli	1 cup	7
Brussel Sprouts	1 cup	10
Cabbage	1 cup	6
Carrots	1 cup	10
Cauliflower	1 cup	5
Celery	1 cup	5
Cucumbers	1 cup	4
Eggplant	1 cup	8
Green pepper	1 cup	6
Greens:		
Turnip	1 cup	5
Spinach	1 cup	4
Mustard	1 cup	6
Beet	1 cup	5
Collards	1 cup	7
Kale	1 cup	7
Lettuce, all varieties	1 cup	2
Okra	1 cup	10
Onions	1 cup	10–15
Parsley	1 cup	trace
Radishes	2 medium	1
Soybeans	1 cup	10
String beans (green & yellow)	1 cup	7
Summer Squash	1 cup	8
Tomatoes, fresh	1 cup	10–15
Turnips	1 cup	8

These carbohydrate values were obtained from *Home and Garden Bulletin #72*, "Nutritive Value of Foods," published by the United States Department of Agriculture, revised April, 1981.

Foods You Can Eat Freely

. . . Unprocessed nuts, seeds, † fats & oils
(Contain little or no carbohydrate)

	Portion	Grams of Carbohydrate
Almonds	¼ cup	6
Brazil nuts	1 ounce	3
Cashews	¼ cup	10
Filberts	¼ cup	5
Pecans	¼ cup	4
Pumpkin seeds	¼ cup	5
Sunflower seeds	¼ cup	7
Walnuts	¼ cup	5
Almond butter	1 tablespoon	3
Cashew butter	1 tablespoon	5
Sesame butter	1 tablespoon	3
Butter		0
Oils, cold-pressed †† safflower, sunflower, linseed and corn oil (obtained from a natural food store)		0

---

†The late Henry Schroeder of Dartmouth College, a recognized authority on trace minerals, commented, "Nuts . . . contain adequate or surplus amounts of all the trace elements; coming from seeds, they contain the elements needed for the growth of the seed until the plant forms roots . . . *The essential trace elements are much more important than the vitamins. They cannot be synthesized, as can the vitamins . . . Without them, life would cease to exist.*" (Schroeder, H. *The Poisons Around Us*, Bloomington Indiana University Press, 1974. Pages 118-119. Published in *Prevention*, July, 1975.)

Although nuts, especially peanuts, often contain mold and may not be tolerated by some individuals, I do not routinely recommend that my patients avoid them unless they cause symptoms. Moreover, Rippon pointed out recently that nuts do not promote the growth of candida. Accordingly, individuals who experience symptoms when they eat nuts do so because of allergy to the nuts or the molds in them (see also page 94).

††These oils contain essential fatty acids and do not contain cholesterol. Two tablespoons should be included in your diet each day.

Foods You Can Eat Cautiously

. . . Fruits‡

	Portion	Approximate Grams of Carbohydrate
Apple	1 small	15
Applesauce, unsweetened	½ cup	12
Apricots, fresh	½ cup	10
Avocado	1 cup	10
Banana	1 medium or ½ cup	26
Berries, fresh or frozen without sugar:		
Blackberries	½ cup	10
Blueberries	½ cup	10
Raspberries	½ cup	10
Strawberries	½ cup	6
Cherries	10	12
Grapefruit	½ grapefruit	13
Grapes	12	12
Lemon	½ lemon	3
Lemon juice	½ cup	10
Mango	½ small	19
Orange	1 small	11–15
Orange juice	1 cup	26
Papaya	½ cup	7
Peach	1 medium	10
Pear	1 medium	22–30
Pineapple	½ cup	11
Plums	1 medium	8

‡ Researcher John W. Rippon, Ph.D., has found that fruits promote yeast growth. (see pages 117-118.)

Foods You Can Eat Cautiously

Breads, Biscuits & Muffins:
All breads listed are made with baking powder or baking soda as the leavening agent. DO NOT USE YEAST. To avoid yeast and to obtain more of the vitamins and minerals your body needs, use whole wheat flour or stone-ground cornmeal. (You'll find *Shopping Tips* and *Food Sources* on pages 85-86.)

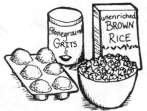

	Portion	Approximate Grams of Carbohydrate
Whole Wheat Biscuit	1 (2" in diameter)	15
Whole Wheat Muffin	1 (2" in diameter)	15
Whole Wheat Pancake	1 (5" in diameter)	15
Popovers	1 (3"x3")	8
Cornbread	1 sq. (2"x2"x1")	15
Corn Muffin	1 sq. (2"x2")	15
Rice Cakes	2	15

Cereals and other grain products:

	Portion	
Barley (pearled)	¼ cup uncooked or 1 cup cooked	36
Cream of Wheat	½ cup cooked	11
Puffed Rice	1 cup	13
Puffed Wheat	1 cup	12
Shredded Wheat	1 biscuit	20
Stoneground Wheat	¼ cup	20
Grits, stoneground, unenriched	½ cup, cooked	13
Brown rice, unenriched	½ cup, cooked	20–25
Oatmeal, long cooking	½ cup, cooked	12
Whole Wheat Cereal	⅓ cup uncooked or ⅔ cup cooked	21
Popcorn (popped)	3 cups	10

Foods You Can Eat Cautiously

High Carbohydrate Vegetables:
(Sugar is added to some canned or frozen vegetables which would make the carbohydrate content even higher.)

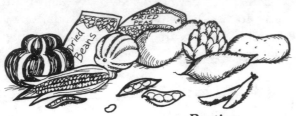

	Portion	Grams of Carbohydrate
Sweet Corn	½ cup	15–25
Lima Beans	½ cup	16–20
English Peas	½ cup	10–15
White Potatoes (baked)	½ lb.	33
Winter squash, acorn, or butternut	½ cup	16
Sweet Potatoes	½ cup	32
Beans and peas, dried and cooked	½ cup	20

Milk:†

Whole Milk or Low Fat Milk	1 cup	11-12

---

† *Many people do not tolerate milk and other dairy products.* Some individuals have a deficiency of the enzyme, lactase, which is needed to digest milk. Others experience problems because they're allergic to milk.

Either whole milk or low fat milk may promote the growth of candida. Here's why: Lactose (milk sugar) is readily converted into glucose and fructose by bacteria and enzymes in the digestive tract. *Accordingly, do not use milk during the early weeks of the low carbohydrate diet.* However, as your immune system improves you may be able to include limited amounts of milk in your diet, especially for use in cooking.

Yogurt is a different story. Unsweetened yogurt you make at home contains quantities of friendly bacteria, Lactobacillus acidophilus, which help crowd out candida from your digestive tract. Yogurt may also be used in the vagina to combat candida. (See page 267 for instructions on making yogurt.)

Low Carbohydrate Diet

Meal Suggestions

BREAKFAST

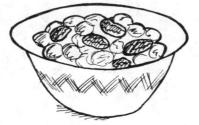

2/3 cup cooked whole wheat cereal (21 grams)
Butter or linseed oil
1/4 cup pecans (4 grams)

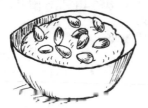

3/4 to 1 cup cooked oatmeal
    with butter (18 to 24 grams)
1/4 cup almonds (6 grams)

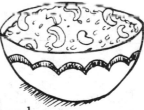

3/4 cup cooked brown rice with butter and
    cashew nuts (24 grams)

References to *grams* in the *Meal Suggestions* refer to grams of carbohydrate.

Low Carbohydrate Diet
Meal Suggestions
BREAKFAST

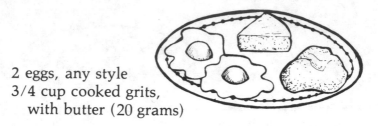

2 eggs, any style
3/4 cup cooked grits,
   with butter (20 grams)

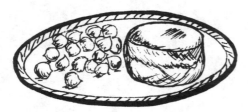

1 or 2 whole wheat biscuits† with
   butter (15 to 30 grams)
1/4 cup filberts (5 grams)

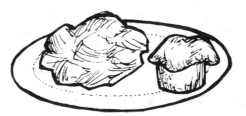

Tuna (water packed)
1 or 2 whole wheat popovers with butter† (8 to 16 grams)

---

† See Recipes, pages 111-116.

Low Carbohydrate Diet
Meal Suggestions
LUNCH

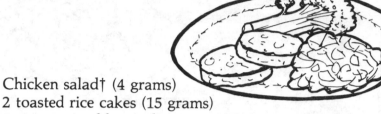

Chicken salad† (4 grams)
2 toasted rice cakes (15 grams)
1 cup steamed broccoli (7 grams)

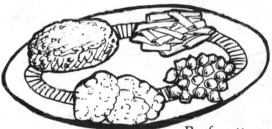

Beef patty
1 cup string beans (8 grams)
1/4 cup filberts (5 grams)
1 cup steamed cauliflower (5 grams)

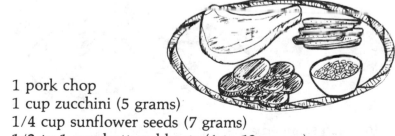

1 pork chop
1 cup zucchini (5 grams)
1/4 cup sunflower seeds (7 grams)
1/2 to 1 cup buttered beets (6 to 12 grams)

---

† See Recipes, pages 111-116.

Low Carbohydrate Diet

Meal Suggestions

LUNCH

Tuna fish with lemon & chopped celery
1/4 cup pecans (4 grams)
Salad with 1/2 tomato, lettuce, green
    pepper, cucumber, radish (5 grams)
Linseed oil & lemon juice dressing
1 or 2 whole wheat popovers (8 to 16 grams)

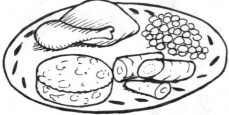

Baked chicken†
1/2 to 1 cup peas & carrots (12 to 24 grams)
1 or 2 toasted rice cakes (7 to 14 grams)

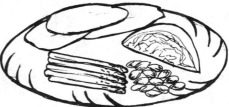

Sliced turkey breast
1/2 to 1 cup steamed asparagus (3 to 6 grams)
1/4 cup almonds (6 grams)
1 cup steamed cabbage

---

† See Recipes, pages 111-116.

Low Carbohydrate Diet
Meal Suggestions
MAIN MEAL

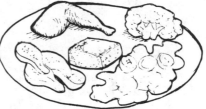

Baked chicken
1/2 cup cauliflower† (3 grams)
1/2 to 1 cup summer squash (4 to 8 grams)
Mixed green salad with linseed oil
   and lemon juice dressing (2 grams)
1 piece corn bread† (15 grams)

Pork chops
1 cup turnip greens (5 grams)
1/2 cup okra† (5 grams)
1/cup raw green pepper strips (3 grams)

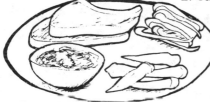

Roast turkey
1/2 cup baked acorn squash† (12 grams)
1 cup steamed spinach (4 grams)
Summertime salad† (5 grams)

---

† See Recipes, pages 111-116.

105

Low Carbohydrate Diet

Meal Suggestions

MAIN MEAL

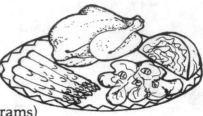

Baked rock cornish hen
1 cup steamed cabbage (6 grams)
1 cup asparagus (6 grams)
Salad with lettuce, (2 grams)
1/4 cup pecans (4 grams)

Sauteed liver† (10 grams)
1/2 cup carrots (5 grams)
1/2 cup raw or steamed broccoli (3 grams)

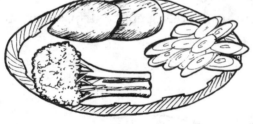

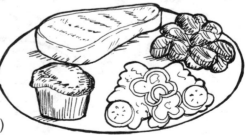

Steak (or hamburger patty)
1/2 to 1 cup eggplant (3 to 6 grams)
Mixed green salad with cucumbers
   and green peppers (3 grams)
Whole wheat popover (8 grams)

---

† See Recipes, pages 111-116.

7-Day Meal Plan

(low carbohydrate)

DAY I
Breakfast
1 cup oatmeal—24 grams.
  with butter
¼ cup almonds—6 grams.

Lunch
Tuna fish
½ whole wheat biscuit
  —15 grams.†
1 small tomato—7 grams.
1 cup lettuce—2 grams.

Dinner
Baked chicken†
½ cup cauliflower—3 grams.
Winter squash—16 grams.†
Corn muffin—15 grams.

Snacks: 1/4 cup pecans—4
  grams
1/2 cup raw carrots—5 grams

DAY II
Breakfast
2 eggs boiled
whole wheat pancakes
  —16 grams.

Lunch
Beef patties
1 whole wheat popover—8 grams
½ cup steamed asparagus
  —3 grams.†
1 cup lettuce—2 grams.
1 cup tomatoes—10 grams

Dinner
Pork chop casserole—30
grams.†
1 toasted rice cake—7 grams
1/4 cup raw carrots—2 grams

Snacks:
1/2 cup celery—3 grams
1/4 cup filberts—5 grams

Caloric requirement can be met with additional protein and fats.

† See Recipes, pages 111-116.

7-Day Meal Plan

(low carbohydrate)

DAY III
Breakfast
⅔ cup whole wheat cereal
  with butter—21 grams.
¼ cup pecans—4 grams.

Lunch
2 or 3 rice cakes—15 to 22 grams.
¼ cup salmon, sunflower seeds
  & sunflower oil—7 grams.

Dinner
Sauteed liver slivers—10 grams.
½ cup steamed carrots—5 grams.
1 cup raw or steamed
  broccoli—8 grams.

Snacks: Whole wheat popover,
  3"x3"—8 grams.†
1/2 cup chopped cabbage with
  linseed and lemon dressing
  —3 grams

DAY IV
Breakfast
½ cup brown rice—17 grams.
  with butter
¼ cup cashews—10 grams.

Lunch
Chicken salad with blender
  mayonnaise—5 grams.†
Corn muffin with butter
  —15 grams.†

Dinner
Meat loaf (¼ of recipe)
  —15 grams.†
½ cup turnip greens—3 grams.
¼ cup peas—10 grams.
1 cup broccoli—7 grams.

Snacks:
¼ cup almonds—6 grams
Radishes—1 to 2 grams

Caloric requirement can be met with additional protein and fats.

---

† See Recipes, pages 111-116.

7-Day Meal Plan

(low carbohydrate)

Day V
Breakfast
2 Scrambled eggs
½ cup cooked grits with
  butter—13 grams

DAY VI
Breakfast
½ cup cooked brown rice
  with butter—20-25 grams
¼ cup cashews—10 grams

Lunch
Fish cakes—10 grams†
½ cup carrots—5 grams

Lunch
Roast beef
½ to 1 potato—12 to 24 grams
Summertime salad—8 grams†

Dinner
Broiled lamb chops
½ to 1 cup zucchini
  —12.5 to 25 grams
3 to 6 radishes—1 to 2 grams
1 corn muffin—15 grams†

Dinner
Baked rock cornish hen
1 cup steamed cabbage
  —6 grams
½ to 1 cup carrots
  —5 to 10 grams

Snacks:
¼ cup pecans—4 grams
½ cup raw carrots—5 grams

Snacks:
½ cup raw broccoli—4 grams
¼ cup pumpkin seeds—5 grams

Caloric requirement can be met with additional protein and fats.

---

† See Recipes, pages 111-116.

7-Day Meal Plan
(low carbohydrate)

DAY VII
Breakfast
Grilled pork chop
½ cup cooked barley
 —18 grams

Lunch
Tuna fish
Whole wheat biscuit with
 butter—15 grams†
¼ cup sunflower seeds
 —7 grams

Dinner
Baked chicken†
1 cup lettuce—2 grams
2 radishes—.7 grams
1 cup tomatoes—4 grams
Spoonbread, 2"x2"—10 grams

Snacks:
⅔ to 1 cup raw cauliflower
 —3 to 5 grams
¼ cup almonds—6 grams

Caloric requirement can be met with additional protein and fats.

_____

† See Recipes, pages 111-116.

13
Yeast-Free Recipes

Swiss Steak
20 grams carbohydrate

2 lbs. round steak, cut into serving
   size pieces
2 tbsp. unrefined vegetable oil

Heat skillet to 375°, add oil, then brown
the meat. Place in casserole and add:

   1 medium onion (½ cup), chopped
   ½ cup chopped celery
   ¼ cup chopped green pepper
   1 cup peeled, chopped fresh
     tomatoes
   ½ cup carrots, sliced
   2 cups water

Cover and bake at 300° for 3-4 hours.
Serves 4.

Meat Loaf
57 grams carbohydrate;
10 per serving

2 lbs. ground beef
1 cup oats, uncooked (old
   fashioned)
1 egg, beaten
¼ cup chopped onion
1 cup water
1 tsp. salt

Combine ingredients. Shape into loaf
and bake in 9 x 5 pan at 350° for about
1 hour. Serves 6.

Sauteed Liver Slivers
50 grams carbohydrate

¼ cup whole wheat flour
¼ cup cold-pressed veg. oil
1 lb. beef liver cut into slivers
1 onion, chopped
Salt to taste

Roll liver slivers in whole wheat flour.
Heat oil in pan. Saute onions and liver.
Salt and serve.

Fish Cakes
40 grams carbohydrate
10 per serving

2 cups tuna fish
1 cup cooked brown rice
1 egg
1 small onion, finely chopped
1 tbsp. lemon juice (fresh)
3 tbsp. melted butter or unrefined
   vegetable oil
1 cup finely ground nuts

Beat egg, add tuna, rice, onion, lemon
juice and oil. Blend well and form into
patties. Roll in nut meal and place on
oiled baking sheet. Bake in 350° oven
about 15 minutes or until brown and
bubbly. May substitute any cooked fish
or poultry for tuna. Makes approximately 8 patties. Serves 4.

Pork Chops and Brown Rice
165 grams carbohydrate;
40 per serving

4 pork chops
1 cup brown rice
2½ cups boiling water
½ cup chopped green pepper
¼ cup chopped onion
½ tsp. salt

Soak rice in boiling water for at least 30-min. Brown pork chops. Set aside. In same frying pan, add remaining ingredients. Simmer 10-min. Pour rice mixture into a oiled baking dish. Layer chops on top. Cover. Bake at 350° for 1 hour. Serves 4.

Baked Chicken
0 grams carbohydrate

Oil bottom of oven-baking dish with a cold-pressed vegetable oil. Lay chicken pieces in pan (skin side down), sprinkle with salt and cover with foil. Bake at 375° for ½ hour. Remove foil, turn pieces, and bake an additional 20 to 30 min., until brown and tender.

Pork Chop Casserole
100 grams carbohydrate;
25 per serving

1-10 oz. package frozen green beans
2 medium onions, sliced
2 or 3 potatoes, peeled and sliced
6 pork chops
salt

Layer beans, onions, potatoes in an oiled 13 x 9 baking pan or casserole. Sprinkle with a bit of salt. Place pork chops on top, cover and bake at 375° for ¾ hour. Remove cover (or foil) and bake an additional 15 min. until chops are tender and brown. Serves 4.

Chicken Salad
5 grams carbohydrate;
1 per serving

2 cups finely chopped cooked chicken
½ cup finely chopped celery
2 to 4 hard cooked, chopped eggs
1 medium onion, chopped

Moisten with blender mayonnaise. Serves 4.

Easy Chicken and Rice
170 grams carbohydrate;
10-12 per serving

3 lbs. frying chicken pieces
1 cup brown rice
2 cups water
½ tsp. salt
1½ tbsp. butter
3 tbsp. chopped fresh parsley
Optional: Onions, celery, green pepper, nuts

Place rice, water, salt, butter and parsley in 4 quart casserole. Stir and bring to a boil. Salt chicken and lay on top of rice. Lower heat to simmer; cover tightly and cook 45 to 60 min. until water is absorbed and chicken is tender.

Barley or Rice Soup
88 grams carbohydrate;
22 per serving

1 - 3 lbs. chicken, disjointed
8 cups cold water
½ cup onion, chopped
1 tbsp. sea salt
½ cup barley or brown rice
1 cup celery, chopped

Place all ingredients in a large pan and cook over medium heat until done. Or, may be cooked all day in a slow cooker. Serves 4.

Best Barley Soup

¼ cup whole barley - cooked in 6 cups of water for 1 hour

Add and cook until tender:
  1 cup carrots
  ½ cup celery
  ¼ cup onions, chopped
  2 cups tomatoes, chopped
  1 cup peas - fresh or frozen

Add fresh parsley just before serving.

Salmon Patties
64 grams carbohydrate
16 per serving

1 lb. salmon with liquid
⅓ cup whole wheat flour
¼ cup stoneground corn meal
¼ cup wheat germ
2 eggs, beaten
½ cup chopped onion
¼ cup chopped bell pepper
1 tbsp. lemon juice
¼ to ½ cup unrefined vegetable oil
  for frying

Flake salmon mashing bones well. Mix all ingredients together. Form into patties. Brown in oil on medium heat for 15 minutes. Serves 4.

Stewed Okra

Okra
Onion
Tomatoes
Corn
Sea salt

Saute okra and onion in a bit of unrefined vegetable oil. Add fresh tomato, fresh or frozen corn, a bit of salt and simmer until tender. May thicken with stoneground corn meal if desired.

Zucchini and Tomatoes

Zucchini
Onion
Tomato
Fresh Parsley

Saute zucchini and onion until tender. Add chopped tomato, continue to stir until cooked. Add parsley and a bit of sea salt and serve.

Green Beans with Almonds

Fresh or frozen green beans
Onion
Unrefined vegetable oil
Fresh parsley
Slivered blanched almonds

Steam green beans until tender. In separate pan saute onion in vegetable oil until tender. Add green beans, parsley and almonds. Sprinkle lightly with salt and serve.

Summertime Salad
20 grams carbohydrate
5 per serving

1 cup cucumber, diced
¼ cup onion, chopped
1 cup tomatoes, diced
½ tsp. sea salt (or less)

NO NEED FOR DRESSING

Serves 4.

Acorn Squash

Cut squash in half and remove seeds. In baking pan place 1 tbsp. unrefined vegetable oil and 1 cup water. Lay halves in pan cut side down and bake in 375° oven for 30 minutes. Turn (face up), brush with oil and sea salt and bake another 20-30 minutes until tender.

Stir Fried Vegetable Scramble

2 tbsp. unrefined vegetable oil or butter
2 tbsp. chopped onion
2 tbsp. chopped green pepper
½ cup fresh chopped tomato
½ to 1 cup cooked vegetables
2 to 4 slightly beaten eggs

Heat skillet, add oil, onions and green pepper. Stir fry until tender. Add tomato and other vegetables. Bring to boil, stirring constantly. Add eggs and cook, stirring gently. Serve immediately.

Wheat Biscuits
180 grams carbohydrate
15 per slice

2 cups whole wheat flour
4 tsps. baking powder·
½ tsp. salt
⅓ cup unrefined vegetable oil
¾ to 1 cup water or milk†

Mix together dry ingredients, add oil and mix well (important). Add enough water to make a soft dough that is not sticky. Mix just enough to moisten dry ingredients. With hands, pat out dough to ¾″ thickness on floured board. Cut with glass. Place on oiled baking sheet and bake 20 minutes or until done in a 450° oven. 12 biscuits.

Blender Mayonnaise

2 eggs at room temperature
2 tbsp. fresh squeezed lemon juice
¼ tsp. sea salt
1¼ cup unrefined vegetable oil

Combine all ingredients except oil in blender at high speed for 1 minute. Slowly add oil. Store in glass jar. Refrigerate.

---

† Milk may be used if tolerated.

Zucchini Florentine

6 small zucchini - ¼ in. slices
2 T. butter
1 cup milk
3 slightly beaten eggs
1 tsp. salt

Put zucchini in 1½ qt. casserole. Dot with butter. Bake at 400° for 15 minutes.

Combine and pour remaining ingredients over zucchini. Set casserole in shallow pan with one inch hot water. Bake 350° for 40 minutes until knife comes out clean.

Whole Wheat Popovers
97 grams carbohydrate
8 per popover

3 eggs
1 cup water or milk†
3 tbsp. butter
1 cup whole wheat flour

Beat eggs until foamy. Add water and butter and continue beating. Add flour and blend. Fill greased muffin cups ⅔ full. Bake at 375° for 50 minutes. Makes 12 popovers.

Banana-Oat Cake
102 grams carbohydrate
11 per piece

2 cups oat flour
¼ tsp. salt
2 tbsp. unrefined vegetable oil
2 tsp. baking powder
½ cup mashed banana
2 eggs
3 tbsp. cold water

Mix dry ingredients. Beat eggs. Add water, oil and mashed banana. Blend with dry ingredients. Bake in 8″x8″ pan at 350° for 25 to 30 minutes. Cut in 9 pieces.

Better Butter

1 stick (½ cup) butter,
  room temperature
½ cup linseed oil

Blend until light and fluffy. Store in glass container. Use as you would regular butter or margarine.

Corn Bread

209 grams carbohydrate
23 per piece

1¾ cups stoneground
  corn meal
⅓ cup whole wheat flour
3 tsp. baking powder
1 tsp. sea salt
1 egg lightly beaten
3 tbsp. cold pressed vegetable oil
1½ cups water or milk†

Combine dry ingredients, beat egg, add oil and water and blend all together. Bake in oiled 8″ square pan 425° 20 to 25 minutes. Cut 9 pieces.

Spoon Bread

90 grams carbohydrate
10 per square

1¼ cups water or milk†
¾ cup stoneground
  cornmeal
¾ tsp. sea salt
3 eggs, separated
3 tbsp. cold pressed vegetable oil

Bring water to boil. Pour in cornmeal and stir constantly and cook until thickened. Add salt and lightly beaten egg yolks and oil. Remove from heat and cool slightly. Fold in stiffly beaten egg whites. Bake in greased 8″ square baking dish at 375° 35 to 40 minutes. Cut in 9 squares.

† Milk may be used if tolerated.

Rice-Oat Pancakes

104 grams carbohydrate

½ cup rice flour
¾ cup Old Fashioned oats - blend
  in blender until fine
1 tbsp. baking powder
¼ tsp. baking soda
2 tbsp. unrefined vegetable oil
½ tsp. sea salt
3 tbsp. apricot puree (or egg)
½ cup Soyquik

Mix all ingredients together and drop tablespoonful onto oiled skillet.

Sunflower Crackers

95 grams carbohydrate

1 cup whole wheat flour
3 tbsp. sunflower seed butter (blend
  speeds in food processor)
2 tbsp. cold pressed vegetable oil
3 tbsp. water
¼ tsp. sea salt

Combine flour, sunflower seed butter and oil. Gradually add water, adding just enough to form a soft dough. Add salt. Knead and roll on floured surface to 1/8″ thickness. Cut in shapes, prick with a fork and bake at 350° for 10 minutes or until browned. Cool.

Oat Griddle Cakes

64 grams carbohydrate

¾ cup cooked Old Fashioned oats
1¼ to 1½ cup milk or water
1 egg
2 tbsp. pressed oil
¾ cup oat flour
1 tsp. baking powder
½ tsp. salt

Mix all ingredients together and spoon onto greased skillet.

115

Potato Pancakes
206 grams carbohydrate
17 per cake

3 cups potatoes, grated raw
1 cup onion, grated
3 eggs, beaten
½ tsp. sea salt
2 tbsp. whole wheat flour
2 tbsp. unrefined vegetable oil

Drop by tablespoonsful on hot oiled skillet. Lower heat slightly and brown, turn and brown other side. Makes 12 pancakes.

Rice Muffins
174 grams carbohydrate

1½ cups rice flour
½ tsp. sea salt
2 tsp. baking powder
¼ tsp. baking soda
4 tbsp. unrefined vegetable oil
3 tbsp. apricot puree
1 cup water or Soyquik

Mix and spoon into greased muffin tins and bake at 350° for 15 to 20 minutes. Makes 12 muffins.

Pancakes
194 grams carbohydrate
8 per 4" cake

1½ to 2 cups water or milk†
2 eggs
2 tbsp. unrefined vegetable oil
3 tsp. salt
2 cups whole wheat flour
2 tsp. baking powder

Beat eggs, add water and oil and blend. Add dry ingredients and blend well. Bake on hot, oiled griddle. makes about 2 dozen 4" cakes.

† Milk may be used if tolerated.

Corn Muffins
183 grams carbohydrate
15 per muffin

1¼ cup whole wheat flour
¾ cup stoneground corn meal
4½ tsp. baking powder
1 tsp. sea salt (optional)
1 egg
⅔ cup water or milk†
⅓ cup unrefined vegetable oil

Sift dry ingredients together. In separate bowl blend egg, water and oil; add to dry mixture and stir with a spoon just enough to dampen all ingredients. Place in 12 greased muffin tins and bake in 425° oven 25 to 30 minutes. Serves 12.

Applesauce Muffins
206 grams carbohydrate
17 per muffin

1 large egg
2 tbsp. unrefined vegetable oil
1½ cups unsweetened applesauce
2 cups whole wheat flour
¾ tsp. baking soda
2 tsp. baking powder
¼ tsp. sea salt

Beat together egg, oil and applesauce. Add flour, soda, baking powder and salt; beat well. Spoon into oiled and floured muffin tins. Bake at 375° for 20 to 25 minutes until firm to touch and browned. Makes 12 muffins.

Wheat-Nut Snack
3 cups shredded wheat bits
3 cups pecans
¼ cup butter, melted

Melt butter in baking pan in 250° oven. Add wheat bits and nuts; mix well and bake 30 to 40 minutes.

14

Fruit-free, Sugar-free, Yeast-free Diet

Helping my candida patients with their diets hasn't been easy for me . . . or for them. And the more I learn about the relationship of diet to human illness, the more excited I become. Yet, sometimes it seems the more I know, the more unanswered questions I have. (see also page 70.)

On December 17, 1983, I interviewed John W. Rippon, Ph.D., of the University of Chicago, an authority on yeasts and molds†. Here's a transcript of our conversation:

Rippon: "Yeasts thrive on the simple carbohydrates. These include cane sugar, beet sugar, honey, corn syrup, maple syrup and molasses. *In addition, eating fruits promotes yeast growth.* Here's why: Fruits are loaded with fructose; in spite of their fiber content, fruits are readily converted to fructose and other simple sugars in the intestinal tract, thereby encouraging the growth of *Candida albicans.*"

Crook: "How about the the grains and the potatoes and the other high carbohydrate vegetables?" Do they promote yeast growth?

Rippon: "No. And I base this opinion on what I know about the nutrition of the yeast organism. (Incidentally, this is well summarized in the book by Frank C. Odds,[3] a British mycologist.)The whole grains are difficult to digest, and whole wheat, brown rice and other whole grains are digested only slowly. Accordingly, they don't seem to be broken down to the point where yeasts can easily ferment them."

---

† Dr. Rippon is the author of the comprehensive 842 page book, MEDICAL MYCOLOGY[2].

There really isn't any experimental evidence I could find on the subject except that grains, by themselves, aren't utilizable by yeasts. This is why, in making beer, you have to predigest the wheat, rice or other grain product using malt which has an enzyme, diastase, in it. So it would seem to me that whole grains would be against the metabolism of yeasts in contrast to the fruits."

Crook: "How about peas, beans and other legumes?"

Rippon: "They don't contain a large percentage of utilizable carbohydrate, so shouldn't cause trouble. To repeat, it's the short chain, utilizable carbohydrates such as those found in sugar, honey, corn syrup, maple syrup and fruits which cause the trouble.

"When you eat fruits, you produce carbon dioxide. We've had patients who so overindulged in fruits and got so gassy that they had to come into the hospital. Gas produced by beans is a different sort of gas. It is methane produced by bacteria rather than carbon dioxide which comes from yeasts.

"White flour products which are easier to break down than whole wheat products may be more conducive to yeast growth than whole grain products."

Crook: "How about mushrooms, Brewer's yeast, moldy cheese and other yeast-containing products which often cause trouble? Do they do this by encouraging the growth of candida?"

Rippon: "No. Eating yeast or mold-containing foods doesn't promote the growth and multiplication of candida. So reactions to yeast-containing foods or beverages must be caused by an allergy to yeast products."

"The Fruit-free, Sugar-Free, Yeast-Free Diet is identical to the *Candida Control Diet* described on pages 75-93, with this exception: *You must avoid all fruits and fruit juices for the first 3 to 6 weeks of your treatment program. Then, if you're doing well, experiment and rotate small amounts of fruit into your diet every fourth day.*

I love fruits and feel they're an important part of a balanced diet. Moreover, many of my patients with yeast-connected health problems have improved during the past several years, even though they continued to eat fruits. But since talking to Dr. Rippon I'm taking a closer look at the role of fruits in causing problems in my patients.

The Yeast-Free, Sugar-Free, Fruit-Free, Grain-Free, Nut-Free, Milk-Free Diet

This is the initial diet recommended (for a period of three weeks) by Shirley Lorenzani, Ph.D. and associates of St. Petersburg, Florida (see also page 71) and by the Price-Pottenger Nutrition Foundation (PPNF) of California‡ (see also page 265). Here's a summary of their dietary instructions:

"Yeast grows on sugar and starch and is fed by gluten-containing grains. Gluten-containing grains include wheat, oats, rye and barley.

"Corn, rice, potatoes and millet may be eaten in very small quantities by most individuals. Some people, however, must temporarily exclude all these starchy foods from the diet.

"Pasteurized milk encourages candida growth. Avoid milk and milk products except sweet butter.

"Nuts accumulate mold and should not be eaten. Eating fruit will boost blood sugar levels and encourage yeast growth. Fruits and fruit juices must be temporarily omitted from the diet.

What is left to eat? Eggs, fish and animal products of all kinds (if the meat is fresh). All vegetables are 'potentially acceptable'. Only starchy ones such as potatoes and sweet potatoes must be avoided by some people."

"Is it possible to eat out?" "Yes! Just order carefully. Skip the cocktails. Have oil and lemon juice on your salad. Order meat, chicken or other animal protein prepared without sauces which might contain sugar, mushrooms, wheat and other harmful ingredients. Broiled or plain items are obviously the safest choice. Steamed vegetables are perfect. Skip bread, crackers and dessert."

---

‡ I visited with Pat Connolly, Curator of PPNF in December, 1983. During our conversation Pat commented,

"We've seen, talked to and heard from thousands of candida victims who have responded to this diet. Included are many who hadn't been helped by other treatment programs.

"In our experience all carbohydrates, especially those found in fruits and milk, promote yeast growth. This is why we feel all fruits and milk must be avoided until the patient improves."

I must admit that I was impressed with the information Pat gave me. Moreover, her views on fruits and milk were recently supported by Rippon and by Dr. John A. Henderson of San Diego (see pages 293-294). However, I am reluctant to recommend a diet which eliminates whole grains and nuts until clinical and laboratory studies show that it is necessary. As I have noted previously, each person—including those with yeast-connected illness—is unique. *So the diet you'll need to use will usually have to be based on trial and error including attention to specific food allergies and intolerances.* (See also pages 67-73, 94, 127-130.)

15

Ideas For Breakfast And Eating On The Run

"Since you *have* to get up, you might as well fix a cheerful breakfast. Not overbearingly cheerful, please! And nothing that requires intricate measuring, sifting, blending or beating . . ."

In her continuing discussion, Janet Lorimer said,

"Experts tell us that breakfast is the most essential meal of the day. It should be nutritious *and* quick-and-easy *and* well balanced *and* appealing to the tastebuds. Studies confirm that children and adults learn and work better when they've eaten breakfast. Unfortunately, breakfast is the most maligned meal of all! Everyone is rushing about in seventeen different directions, and eating seems to be *one* thing no one wants to spend time doing. So, how can you possibly make breakfast your favorite meal against those odds?

"Plan ahead! Spend a few moments the night before planning tomorrow's first meal. Who likes to think about breakfast at 10:30 at night? But it beats staggering into the kitchen the next morning totally unprepared."

Janet's article gives many other suggestions, including making a list of menu ideas, glamorizing the table setting, making your own mixes and freezing for the future.

In discussing these, she commented,

"Never underestimate the power of your freezer to work breakfast miracles. If all you have in your freezer is frozen pizza and two bags of ice cubes, you're not using a valuable ally!"

"When fruit goes on sale, buy in bulk and freeze, following the proper freezing instructions in your cookbook! Frozen fruits lose their crispness

---

† Adapted from the article, "How to Make Breakfast Your Favorite Meal," by Janet Lorimer which was published in the March, 1983 issue of *Bestways Magazine* (pages 43-44). Used with permission.

when they're thawed, but they make a delicious hot compote. There's nothing quite so much fun as eating summer fruit in the dead of winter."

Although all of the "goodies" Janet talks about can't be used on your diet, special yeast free breads can be baked ahead of time and frozen. When you want to use them just reheat in a moderate oven.

For snacks, lunch or eating on the run, you can fill a "brown bag" with hard boiled eggs, raw vegetables and fruits, nuts, rice cakes or meat and bread from your freezer.

16

If Sugar Is A "No-No," What Can I Use?

If candida plays a role in causing your health problems, avoid sugar, because sugar seems to feed the yeast germ and hundreds of my patients have reported,

"When I eat sugar, my symptoms flare up."

Sugar may also trigger symptoms in individuals who do not have candida-related illness.

Yet, because sweetened foods taste good, I'm sure you'd like to know other ways that you can safely sweeten your foods and beverages. Here are comments on sweeteners you may have considered, including some you can use and other which aren't recommended:

Aspartame: In July, 1981, the Food and Drug Administration finally gave its approval for use of a new low calorie sweetener. This product is 200 times sweeter than sugar, but contains only 1/8th the calories found in sugar. The product tastes like sugar, but contains no saccharine or other artificial sweetener.

Aspartame can be found on supermarket shelves across the country under the brand name Equal® or Nutra-Sweet®.

Aspartame was discovered in 1965 when a chemist wet his finger to pick up a piece of paper and noticed a sweet taste. The two compounds he was working with were aspartic acid and the amino acid, phenylalanine (found in proteins). Although neither of these compounds alone taste sweet, combined they're very sweet.

Since the discovery of this product, more than 100 scientific tests for its safety have been conducted during the last 15 years. In addition, scientists at Searle Consumer Products (which markets Equal®) have conducted many formal and impromptu consumer taste tests with men, women and children. These results show that aspartame could be widely accepted as a sugar substitute.

How about safety? Most scientists feel aspartame is safe, since it's made of two normal food ingredients (amino acids) which have been joined together. So when it goes into your body, it's like a tiny bit of food, rather than a synthetic chemical.†

One packet of Equal® has the sweetness of two teaspoons of sugar, but supplies only 4 calories. It costs about 4 cents per packet, so it's much more expensive than saccharin. Also, it can't be used in baking because high heat for long periods of time cause chemical changes in the amino acids, eliminating the sweet taste.

Saccharin: Foods and beverages containing saccharin must be labeled with the following warning:

> "Use of this product may be hazardous to your health. This product contains saccharin which has been determined to cause cancer in laboratory animals."

In spite of this label, I prefer saccharin to sugar, and when used in limited quantities, I feel it is relatively safe. Moreover, a study in a leading medical journal comparing patients with bladder cancer to a similar group who had no cancer, showed no evidence that the cancer patients had consumed more saccharin than those who did not have cancer.

Fruits: Some of my patients with yeast-connected illness tolerate complex carbohydrates, including apples, bananas and pineapple. If you are such a person, Karen Barkie's cookbook, *Sweet and Sugar Free*, (St. Martin's Press, New York, N. Y.) should interest you. It's full of recipes for sugar-free, fruit-sweetened foods.

Other of my patients develop symptoms when they eat fruits. For example, Ted F., a patient with MS who was doing well, was in for a follow-up visit on April 22, 1983. Ted commented,

> "I'm doing great. No symptoms unless I eat yeast-breads or sugar. These foods trigger numbness and weakness, and a large banana will do the same thing. And 39-year-old Lynn, a patient with fatigue, depression and abdominal symptoms, commented, "Grains and fruits of all kinds make my symptoms worse."

---

† R. J. Wurtman recently reported that undesirable effects may occur if large amounts of aspartame are ingested. (New England Journal of Medicine, vol. 309: pages 429-430, August 18, 1983) (For a further discussion of aspartame, see pages 295-296).

Because fruits promote yeast growth, I now tell my patients to avoid them—especially during the first month of their treatment program.

Honey: Many people like honey. And honey is sweeter than sugar. Moreover, over the years, many parents of hyperactive children have reported,

"Sugar makes my child hyperactive, yet he can take honey."

Nevertheless, if your illness is related to candida, stay away from honey . . . at least until your health problems are well controlled. Here's why: Honey resembles sugar in many ways and tends to feed the yeast organism.

Fructose or high Fructose Corn Syrup: This substance has received a great deal of publicity. It's sweeter than cane and beet sugar in cold liquids and is now used in many commercially sweetened foods.

Is it better or safer for you than ordinary table sugar? No, because it feeds the yeast germ just as much as ordinary sugar. Also, it's a lot more expensive.

17

Food Allergies

Reactions to foods have been recognized by numerous observers for many centuries. For example, as early as the 1st century, B.C., Lucretius commented,

> "What is food to one may be fierce poison to others." And perhaps the first report of the use of an elimination diet can be found in the Bible in the first chapter of the Book of Daniel (1:12—15).

Hippocrates[15] also commented,

> " . . . There are certain persons who cannot readily change their diet with impunity; and if they make any alteration in it for one day, or even for a part of a day, are greatly injured thereby. Such persons, provided they take dinner when it is not their wont, immediately become heavy and inactive, both in body and mind, and are weighed down with yawning, slumbering, and thirst; . . . to many this has been the commencement of a serious disease, when they have merely taken twice in a day the same food which they have been in the custom of taking once."

Although scattered references can be found on the relationship of food and food odors to physical symptoms during the past several centuries, it wasn't until about 100 years ago that physicians began to pay attention to what was then called "food idiosyncrasy."

During the current century, thousands of physicians have made clinical observations on the relationship of foods to a wide variety of clinical syndromes and several hundred reports of such food-related reactions can be found in the medical literature.

In spite of these numerous reports, many allergists ignore food-induced reactions and say in effect, "If you can't establish an immunologic mechanism you can't term such reactions allergy." But growing numbers of individuals, including physicians in practice as well as in academic centers, are now recognizing that food-related reactions are common. And one academician commented,

"It will be a long time before we understand all aspects of food allergy; certainly it will not happen in our lifetime."

Obvious Food Allergies: Such allergies are usually caused by uncommonly eaten foods such as shrimp, lobster, cashew nuts or strawberries. However, they can also be caused by peanuts, eggs and other common foods. Individuals with obvious food allergies will show positive reactions to various immunological tests, including the scratch or prick test and the RAST test. By contrast, such tests are usually negative in individuals with hidden food allergies.

Hidden Food Allergies: During the past 27 years, I've found that food-induced reactions have caused health problems in thousands of my patients. And because the foods causing the patients' symptoms are rarely suspected, I've termed these reactions "hidden food allergies."

Such allergies are caused by foods a person eats every day, including especially milk, corn, wheat, egg, sugar, chocolate, citrus and food colors, flavors and additives. They usually develop gradually over a period of weeks, months and years. A person tends to become "addicted" to the foods causing his symptoms. So he's apt to crave them. Symptoms caused by hidden food allergies include fatigue, nasal congestion, dark shadows under the eyes (allergic "shiners"), headache, abdominal pain, muscle and joint pains, bladder symptoms and nervous system symptoms of all types.

Experiences of Other Physicians: Hundreds of other physicians, including Dr. Elmer Cranton of Troutdale, Virginia, Dr. Harold Hedges of Little Rock, Arkansas, and Dr. Doris Rapp of Buffalo, New York, have also found that hidden allergies to common foods often cause chronic and often disabling symptoms in their patients. And Dr. Cranton commented,

"In addition to prescribing nystatin , I nearly always prescribe Elimination Diet A in your book, *Tracking Down Hidden Food Allergy.*[13] This enables me to identify trouble-making foods and remove them from the diet. And by decreasing the patient's allergy load, my overall treatment program is more apt to be successful."

In carrying out Elimination Diet A, the patient avoids milk, egg, wheat, corn, sugar, chocolate, citrus fruits, along with the food colors, dyes and most of the packaged and processed foods. The elimination phase of the diet usually lasts about a week or until there is convincing improvement in symptoms which continues for 48 hours. Then foods are returned to the diet, one food per day, and reactions are noted. By using this diet, I'm able to identify trouble-making foods and remove them from the diet.

And in a Letter to the Editor in the January, 1982 issue of *The Journal of the Arkansas State Medical Association,* Dr, Harold Hedges commented,

> "The longer I practice medicine, the more I'm convinced that many illnesses are caused by what we eat, drink and breathe.
>
> "Since 1963, I've treated many patients with diseases and disorders which I could neither see with the naked eye nor help. Included among these that I label in good faith are patients with tension headache, chronic fatigue, chronic ear problems, sinusitis, irritable colon, depression, anxiety, hyperactivity, nervous stomach and hypochrondriasis. And when I couldn't find another cause, I'd even lay the blame on the poor lowly virus . . . I thank God for viruses, even if I couldn't prove it so, the patient couldn't prove me wrong."

Dr. Hedges has found similar success in using elimination diets. And in a recent conversation with me, he said,

> "I usually use the 'cave man diet' from your book, *Tracking Down Hidden Food Allergy*[13], in working with my adult patients. And this more comprehensive diagnostic diet has enabled me to identify sensitivity to beef, pork, chicken, soy and other foods usually recommended for candida patients. And by identifying these foods and eliminating them, my treatment results are significantly improved."

Rotated Diets: In spite of the gaps which remain in our understanding of food-related problems, countless observers, dating from the time of Hippocrates, have noted that variety or diversity in selecting one's foods lessens a person's chances of developing food-induced reactions. And during the past decade, many individuals, including physicians (and other professionals) and allergy sufferers, have found they can tolerate trouble-making foods and experience fewer symptoms if they rotate their diet.

Rotated Diets

Day	1	2	3	4	5
Meats	Beef	Chicken	Shrimp	Pork	Trout
Fruits	Orange	Banana	Pineapple	Grape	Apple
Vegetables	White potato	Sweet potato	Carrot	Squash	Peas, beans or other legumes
Grains	Wheat	Oats	Rice	Barley	Corn

Karen Dilatush commented,

129

"I began having severe problems from eating the same *good* foods over and over. I improved as soon as I began rotating my diet."

In rotating your diet, you eat a food only once every 4 to 7 days. For example, in rotating fruits, you'd eat oranges on Monday, bananas on Tuesday, apples on Wednesday and pineapple on Thursday. Then on Friday you could start over again with oranges. The same system can be used with other food groups, including meats, vegetables and grains.

Further information about rotated diets can be found in a number of reference books, including "Today's Tuesday, It Must Be Chicken", by Natalie Golos (available from Dickey Enterprises, 635 Gregory Road, Fort Collins, Colorado 80524) and the "Cookbook/Guide to Eating for Allergy", by Virginia Nichols (available from 3350 Fair Oaks Drive, Xenia, Ohio 45385).

Section C

Keeping Candida under control requires more than medication and a special diet.

A number of concepts, drawings and charts in this section have been adapted and modified from material published by

Sidney M. Baker, M.D.

Introduction

18

My grandfather was a country doctor who started practicing medicine in West Tennessee over 100 years ago. My father followed in his footsteps and joined him in practice around 1900. They were both "people doctors" who tried to help their patients with the limited resources available to them at the time. No x-rays, no antibiotics; no polio vaccine; no corticosteroids; no birth control pills; no endoscopic examination; no CAT scans; no cataract or open heart surgery and no hip replacements. No renal dialyses or exchange transfusions; no heart or kidney transplants.

In medicine, just as in transportation, communication and every other area of our lives, changes have been amazing, fantastic and breath-taking. And because of these advances in medicine, many lives have been saved and much suffering relieved.

When my oldest daughter was 4 years old, she developed severe peritonitis following a ruptured appendix. Antibiotics saved her life. And my mother-in-law, who had a total hip replacement when she was 80, kept driving her car and walking a mile a day until she was 90.

Countless numbers of my patients enjoy healthy, productive lives because medical science provided new answers and new therapies.

To cope with the explosion in medical knowledge during the past several decades, medicine has become more highly specialized. Not long ago I visited John Lingo, a medical school classmate. John, an ophthalmologist, practices with a group of nine eye specialists in Mobile, Alabama. As we toured his clinic, Dr. Lingo commented,

"Dr. A. specializes in blepharoplasty (taking tucks in eyelids of people who want to look younger). Dr. B specializes in diseases of the cornea; Dr. C specializes in the retina, and Dr. D specializes in the parts in between!"

133

Similar specialization has taken place in internal medicine, pediatrics, surgery and other areas of medicine. And during the last 10 years, all sorts of new specialists and subspecialists have entered practice in my town and in communities across the country. Many doctors specialize in treating only one part of the body or only one type of disease. Some specialize in treating arthritis or thyroid disease while others specialize in diseases of the digestive tract. Still others specialize in treating headaches, psoriasis, hyperactivity or multiple sclerosis.

With the great increase in medical knowledge, medical education has increasingly stressed the importance of correct diagnosis. Accordingly, great emphasis has been placed on the naming of diseases. Then once a disease is identified and labeled, a treatment plan is established which usually includes drugs or surgery. Without question, such diagnosis and treatment is effective in coping with many contemporary health problems, ranging from acute bacterial meningitis to gallstones.

But is this a perfect answer for every medical problem? Suppose you "feel like the devil" and you undergo a variety of medical examinations and learn that you don't have a "disease?" No brain tumor; no diabetes; no tuberculosis; no gallstones; no appendicitis; no anemia; no "nothing." What then?

This was Marilyn's problem. Marilyn, a 38-year-old professional, enjoyed a happy marriage and a successful career. Moreover, her two youngsters were bright and healthy and added to the happiness of her family. *Her only problem: She rarely felt good.*

Because of premenstrual tension, abdominal pain and menstrual irregularities, Marilyn usually went to her gynecologist for medical care. However, when her headaches became almost incapacitating, she was referred to a neurologist who carried out a variety of tests, including EEG studies and brain scans. Both were said to be "normal."

Then because of recurrent abdominal pain, bloating and other digestive symptoms, Marilyn was referred to a gastroenterologist. After upper and lower GI x-rays, gallbladder x-rays and endoscopic examinations, she was told, "All of your studies are normal." But because of continued abdominal pain and occasional urinary tract infections, she was cystoscoped and kidney x-rays were carried out. These studies were also normal.

Finally, because no "disease" could be identified and she continued to feel tired and depressed, Marilyn's gynecologist suggested that she talk to clinical psychologist, Cheryl Robley, Ph.D. After two visits, Cheryl called me saying,

> "I'd like for you to see Marilyn and see if you can help her with her fatigue and depression. She has no significant psychological hangups and I feel her symptoms are yeast connected."

After taking nystatin and changing her diet, Marilyn improved. She improved even more when she really worked on her diet and avoided all junk foods and began taking yeast-free vitamins and minerals. Further improvement followed the banning of odorous colognes and perfumes, insecticides, bathroom chemicals and other chemical pollutants from her home. Marilyn and her husband, John, have also been taking out more time for exercise, rest and relaxation and Marilyn feels that taking essential fatty acids in the form of linseed oil helps her get rid of her premenstrual tension.

In talking to the patients who come to see me seeking help for yeast-connected illness, here's what I tell them:

1. I possess no "quick fix." No magic pill. Yet, I'll do my best to help you get rid of your symptoms and regain your health.
2. Each person differs from every other person. And I do not think of the "yeast problem" as a disease. Instead, it's only one factor which plays a role in causing your health problems. Other important factors include the quality of the food you eat, the air you breathe, the water you drink and the relationship you enjoy with your family and friends.

So to overcome yeast-connected health problems, we have to take a comprehensive approach. This means you need to understand the many factors that play a role in making you sick and take control of them. Then you can help your own immune system conquer them.

19

To Overcome Candida And Enjoy Good Physical, Mental And Emotional Health:

You Must Seek These Vital Nutrients

Good food provides calories and many other essential substances your body needs to function properly. Proteins, carbohydrates (starches) and fats or oils provide the calories. When they're obtained from good sources, they also furnish your body with essential "micronutrients," including vitamins and minerals.

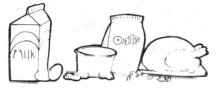

Proteins: Found in meat, fish, eggs, dairy products, nuts & seeds, whole grains, peas and beans (& other vegetables to a lesser extent). Proteins are made up of substances called "amino acids." There are 22 of these and many of them are essential. You increase your chances of good health if you obtain your proteins from a wide variety of sources.

Carbohydrates or starches: There are two types of these; the *"complex" carbohydrates* (found in a wide variety of vegetables, fruits and whole grains), and the *"refined" carbohydrates* found especially in refined sugar and white flour. Although both types of carbohydrates furnish energy, only the complex carbohydrates provide the vitamins and minerals needed for their proper utilization.

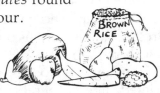

Fats & oils: Limited amounts of these nutrients are an important part of your diet. Yet, there are "good" fats and "bad" fats. The good

fats are the *essential fatty acids* ("EFA's"), including linoleic acid and linolenic acid (obtained especially from unprocessed vegetable oils, including linseed, sunflower, safflower, corn and primrose oils).
They play an important role in many of your body's biochemical processes, including the manufacture of prostaglandins and the strengthening of your immune system.

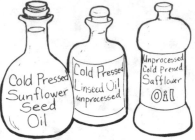

The bad fats include hydrogenated or partially hydrogenated vegetable oils and fats obtained from animal products. Although such fats provide calories, they appear to play a role in plugging up your arteries, leading to the premature development of degenerative disorders.

Other nutrients include iron, calcium and magnesium which are necessary for many vital body functions, including the prevention of anemia, the promotion of strong teeth and bones, a sound heart and a properly functioning nervous system.

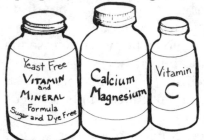

You also need other *"micronutrients"* (*micro* means very small), including both vitamins and minerals. According to the late Dr. Henry Schroeder[16] of Dartmouth College, there are 37 micronutrients, including vitamins A, B-1, B-2, B-3, B-6, B-12, C & D, and the trace minerals, zinc, selenium, chromium, and many others.

Without these micronutrients, your body machinery simply doesn't work well. For example, a zinc deficiency interferes with normal taste, growth and resistance to infection. If you don't get enough chromium, you cannot properly metabolize carbohydrates. Without sufficient vitamin B-6, prostaglandin synthesis is impaired and calcium deficiency renders the white blood cells incapable of making substances they need to kill candida. These are only a few of the hundreds (or even thousands) of important interactions in the body which require micronutrients.

Iron appears to be especially important to people with yeast-related illness. Studies by Higgs & Wells[17] and others suggest that some individuals, even those who aren't anemic, may require iron supplements. Calcium and magnesium supplements are particularly important in young women, especially those of slender build who do not consume dairy products. Without an adequate calcium intake, bones lose their minerals and women, especially those past the menopause, develop osteoporosis.[18a,b,c] This condition weakens the bones, leading to collapsed vertebrae, pinched nerves, broken hips and other disabling health problems.

and you must avoid

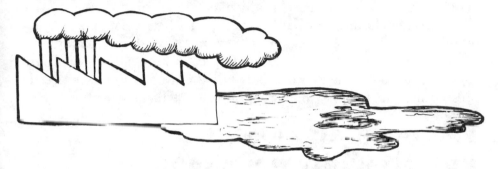

poisons and pollutants of all kinds including those which contaminate the air, soil and water.

Toxic or poisonous substances: Lead from many sources, including leaded gasoline, is polluting our planet. Evidence of such lead pollution can be found in the north polar ice cap which contains much more lead than the south pole, the difference being fewer auto mobiles in the southern hemisphere.

Other toxic minerals include cadmium and mercury. There's also growing evidence that we're ingesting aluminum in many processed foods as well as in foods wrapped in aluminum foil, aluminum in drinking water, aluminum cans and cooking utensils. Although aluminum doesn't appear to be a major environmental poison, it would appear prudent to lessen your exposure to it.

Insecticides and weed killers: These chemicals, sprayed on our fields and farms and in our homes, get into the water supply and into the food chain. And all of us now have DDT and similar poisons in our bodies.

Other chemicals: A variety of other industrial chemicals have been introduced into our environment which are causing health problems in many persons. Substances such as PCB's (polychlorinated biphenyls) have gotten into our soil and water and into the food chain, and have made their way into our bodies. Moreover, human breast milk contains these toxins and pollutants to a degree that concerns many people.

Home chemicals: Our clothing, homes, cosmetics, soaps, deodorants and detergents contain many toxic or potentially toxic chemicals, including formaldehyde, petrochemicals, phenol and many other substances which may accumulate and overload our immune system, increasing our susceptibility to illness. (Recent studies suggest that T-cells and other parts of the immune system are depressed in patients with illness caused by chemical sensitivity.)

you must also avoid nutritionally poor food especially sugar, white flour and hardened vegetable oil

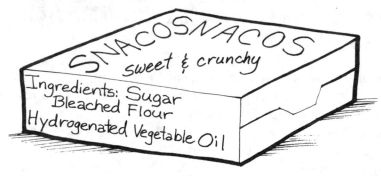

You are what you eat. And if you load up on poor quality foods, including especially foods containing sugar, white flour and hardened vegetable oil, you won't enjoy good health.

Studies by Cheraskin[19] of the University of Alabama which indicates that diets high in refined sugar impair the function of the body's phagocytes (germ-eating white blood cells) which play an important role in resisting bacterial infection.

Studies by Schroeder[16] (and many others) clearly indicate that when whole wheat flour is refined, many essential nutrients are removed, including vitamins and minerals. Included among these are B-vitamins, magnesium, zinc and selenium. Moreover, even when white flour is "enriched" by the addition of a few nutrients, it still lacks other nutrients which are equally essential.

Research by Horrobin and Rudin[20a, b c, & d] shows that diets containing hardened vegetable oil found in many processed and packaged foods may be deficient in essential fatty acids. Such diets may interfere with the formation of prostaglandins E-1 (PGE-1). This, in turn, depresses T-lymphocytes which (as previously mentioned) play an important role in resisting allergies and infections.

Their research also suggests that diets deficient in essential vitamins, trace minerals, essential fatty acids and other nutrients lessen the integrity of the immune system.

you must be treated for
... allergies caused by inhalants
and foods

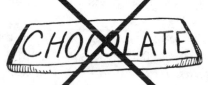
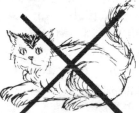

and infections caused
by harmful
microorganisms

Allergies: Many people are troubled by adverse or allergic reactions to substances which do not appear to bother the average person. Such substances include pollens, molds, dust, animal danders, and foods. A number of observers now feel that individuals who react to substances in their diet or environment experience such reactions because their immune system is depressed by poor nutrition and an overload of environmental chemicals.

Many of my patients with food and chemical sensitivities improve and their allergies lessen when they take nystatin and follow a comprehensive program of management. Yet others, especially patients with inhalant allergy, may require allergy testing, followed by the use of allergy extracts, in order to achieve maximum improvement.

Infections caused by harmful micro-organisms, including bacteria, viruses and yeasts (and invasion by parasites). The healthy body with its marvelous immune system and other protective forces, both known and unknown, is usually able to resist or overcome invasion by many such organisms. Yet, when we pollute our environment or eat a poor diet, or upset our body balance with prolonged courses of drugs (including antibiotics and birth control pills), our immune system becomes depressed and these organisms can enter.

For example, when you take a diet high in refined carbohydrates, yeast germs proliferate. And increased numbers of yeast germs put out toxins which depress your immune system and increase your susceptibility to food and chemical allergies, infections, and other illnesses.

Naturally, if you develop a strep throat, bacterial pneumonia or meningitis, you'll need an antibiotic drug. But most of the time, if you run a fever, the cause will be a virus. And if you'll use the "watch and wait" system, plus extra vitamin C and a sugar-free diet, your own immune system will marshal its forces and conquer many invading enemies. Pauling[21] has recently pointed out that large doses of vitamin C will also help you overcome many viral infections.

You Need A Favorable Environment

Sunlight and/or skylight: In appropriate amounts (not too little and not too much) sunlight and other full spectrum light provide vitamin D and other essentials needed for proper growth of plants, animals and humans. (Further information on the importance of full spectrum light can be found in the writings of John Ott. See page 279 for reference.)

Fresh air. You must have fresh air (including oxygen) in order to live.

Pure water. Without water, you cannot survive. And the purer and less polluted the water, the better it is for you.

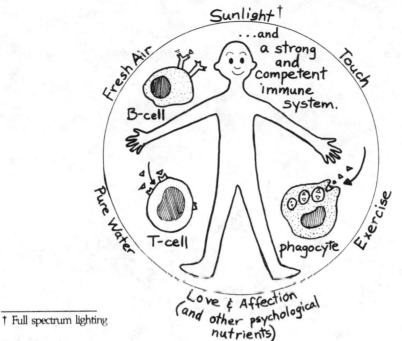

Sunlight †

...and a strong and competent immune system.

Fresh Air

Touch

B-cell

Pure Water

T-cell

phagocyte

Exercise

Love & Affection (and other psychological nutrients)

† Full spectrum lighting

Exercise. Absolutely essential for proper function of your body, including not only your bones and muscles, but also your heart, lungs, brains, and immune system.

Love & Affection. All human beings require affection from the moment of birth throughout life. You must feel accepted, loved, respected and valued for what you are. Without love and affection, you cannot thrive.

Touch. Many recent scientific studies show that touch stimulates the production of hormones and body chemicals, including endorphins which play an important role in your overall health.

A competent and properly functioning immune system: Your immune system resembles your army, navy and marines. It protects you from foreign invaders, including bacteria, viruses, yeasts and chemicals. Some of your defenders are called phagocytes (phago = to eat; cyte = cell). These cells gobble up strep germs, pneumonia germs and other threatening invaders and help you overcome an infection.

Other defenders in your immune system include B-cells and T-cells. These make immunoglobulins of several types which block or neutralize invaders and help the phagocytes and other body defenders protect you. (See, also, pages 163-166.)

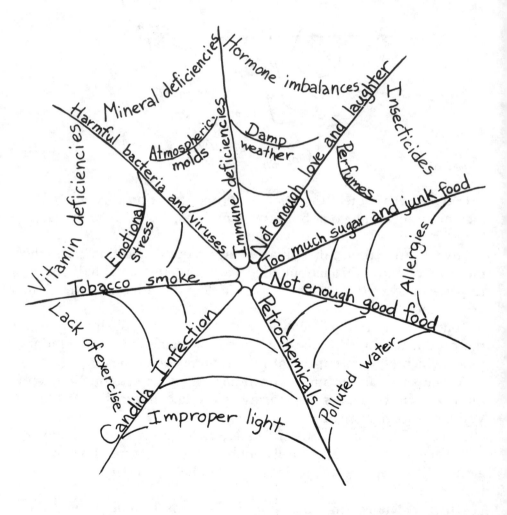

20
The Causes Of Illness Resemble A Web

When you don't feel well, there's always a reason (or many reasons). Some of these are obvious; yet others may be hard to find. Moreover, when you become ill, *your illness is nearly always caused by a web of interacting factors,* rather than a single cause. Although Candida albicans may play an important role in making you sick, to get well and stay well you'll need to pay attention to other factors.

In so doing, you must eat good food, stay away from junk, and make your environment a favorable one. So you'll need fresh air, appropriate lighting (indoors and outdoors) and pure water. You must also avoid or limit your exposure to the many chemicals which are polluting our environment.

Finally, you must receive liberal quantities of "psychological vitamins," including an affectionate, caring relationship with those with whom you live and work.

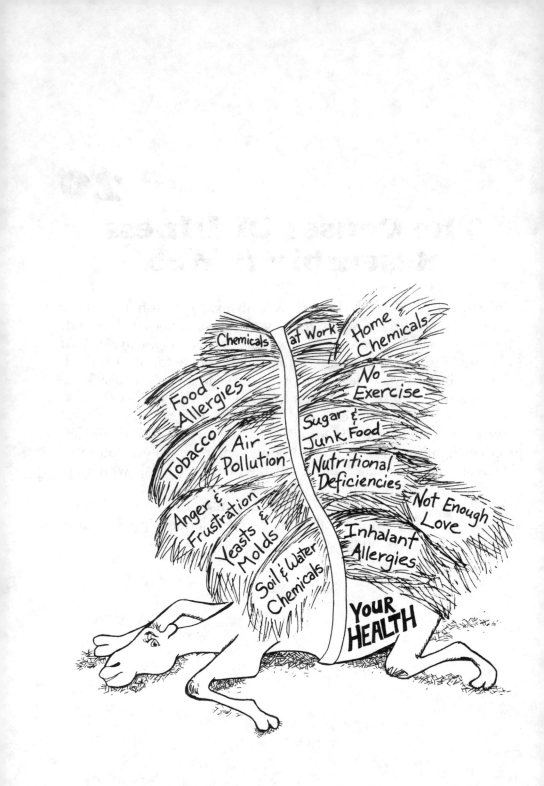

21

Is Your Camel's Load Too Heavy?

If you suffer with severe and persistent allergies and other chronic health problems it may be because of the heavy load of many different things that bother you plus poor nutrition. Rarely is there a single cause. So unloading as many "bundles of straw" as possible is the best way to get the camel (your health) back on its feet.

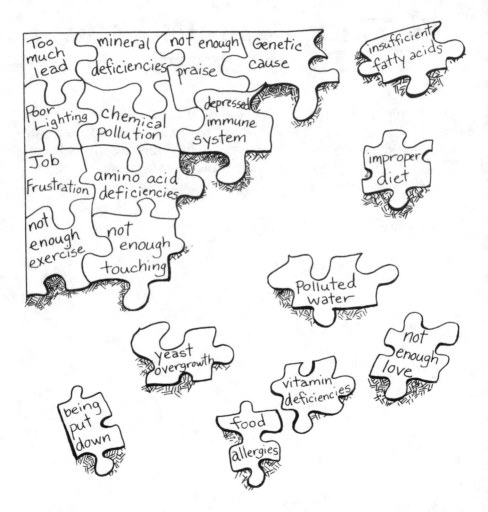

Adapted from Carl Pfeiffer, Ph.D., M.D. Used with permission.

22

The Puzzle
Of Chronic Illness

During the past three years, I've treated over 400 patients with chronic health problems related to "the yeast connection." And although nystatin and diet played an important role in helping most of these patients, many did not improve until other pieces of the puzzle were appropriately treated. (See also pages 232-236.) Examples:

A 40-year-old school teacher felt much worse on damp, muggy days. A room dehumidifier and ionizer helped her symptoms. Control of mold growth in the home played an important role in contributing to the improvement of many other patients.

A 34-year-old mother of four, with candida related health problems, was improving slowly. When blood studies showed a low blood vitamin A level, she was given digestive enzymes and additional vitamin A. Within a short time, she began to show more rapid improvement.

A 16-year old with severe systemic and nervous system symptoms, including peculiar "seizures," was found to be sensitive to a number of common foods he was eating every day. Eliminating these foods and carrying out other parts of a comprehensive program of management resulted in significant improvement.

A 42-year-old secretary suffered from chronic hives, fatigue, depression and mental confusion. Her hives and mental confusion disappeared on treatment with diet and nystatin. A series of vitamin B-12 injections helped relieve her fatigue.

A 4-year-old with recurrent rhinitis, ear problems and irritability improved on diet, nystatin and nutritional supplements. Yet, rhinitis continued until a foam rubber pillow and rubber-stuffed dolls were removed from the child's bed.

Many of my patients continued to be bothered by headaches,

rhinitis, cough, burning eyes and other symptoms until tobacco smoke, insecticides, furniture polishes, colognes and other odorous or "outgassing chemicals" were removed from their homes. Other patients improved when they began drinking filtered water.

Improvement in many patients occurred when essential fatty acids in the form of linseed oil or primrose oil were added to their treatment programs. Still others improved when their inhalant and food allergies were treated with allergy vaccines and extracts.

23
Chemicals May Play A Role In Making You Sick

Margaret, a 58-year-old housewife, came to my office in January, 1983. Here are excerpts from a letter she sent in before her visit:

"In my thirties, I developed post nasal drainage which irritated my throat. The doctors blamed it on 'sinus' and gave me antibiotics which didn't help. Later I read about allergies and experimented with my diet. My symptoms improved when I left off milk.

"At age 39, I gave birth to my fourth child and developed inner ear trouble with dizziness, nausea and vomiting. I was treated by a head specialist with various medications, including antibiotics. I was allergic to all of them. Through further experimentation, I learned I felt better, with less dizziness and heart palpitations, when I left off corn, sweets, dairy products and eggs.

"At the age of 53, I developed stiff and aching joints and began to notice that tobacco smoke, cosmetics, cleaners, paints, dyes and printing ink would bother me. More recently, I've developed reactions to polyester and had to quit crocheting and quilting because I coughed so much when I worked with them."

Margaret was put on a comprehensive treatment program, including nystatin and a yeast free, sugar free diet. She was also tested for a number of foods and given food extracts.

On February 18, 1983, Margaret wrote,

"I feel so much better; it's like I died and went to heaven. I'm still sensitive to chemical fumes and odors so I decided to stay away from church and public places for awhile to avoid these reactions."

On March 22, 1983, Margaret reported,

"I'm still improving, although slowly in some ways. My chemical sen-

151

sitivity is still bad. It seems I find more things in my house each day that bother me. I'm trying to get rid of them but it seems to be an endless task.

"I'm continuing my rotating diet, along with vitamins and primrose oil. My dry skin has improved tremendously and my feelings of depression and uneasiness are also much improved. I'm able to sleep most nights without problems. I'm grateful to you for helping me. Thank you so much."

Like Margaret, many of my patients with yeast connected health problems develop symptoms when they're exposed to diesel fumes, colognes, perfumes, formaldehyde, insecticides, laundry detergents, polyester clothing and other chemicals. *If you suffer from a yeast related illness, learn as much as you can about chemicals and how to avoid them.*

Some chemicals are normally present in your body, including sodium chloride (salt), potassium, calcium and magnesium. They're "normal chemicals" and aren't the ones you need to worry about. Instead, pay attention to "foreign chemicals," especially those derived from petroleum and related sources. These include:

Gasoline	Coal burning stoves	Inks
Natural gas	Brass, metal or shoe polish	Carbon paper
Diesel fumes	Floor waxes	Typewriter stencils
Garage fumes	Wax candles	Clothing dyes
Cleaning fluids	Car roofs & roads	Cosmetics
Nail polish	Asphalt pavements	Disinfectants
Formaldehyde	Furniture polishes	Marking pencils

Others include:

Phenol derivatives (carbolic acid or Lysol®), alcohols, defoliants, and household detergents.

Rubber, including sponge rubber, from rubber pillows, typewriter pads, rubber-base paints, rubber tires, automobile accessories.

Plastics, including plastic upholstery, pillow covers, shoe bags, handbags, plastic folding doors, plastic cement, adhesive tapes.

Synthetic textiles, including dacron, orlon, polyester, rayon, etc.

Paints, varnishes, shellacs, window cleaning fluids, banana oil, ammonia fumes, moth balls, insect repellants, termite exterminating materials, insecticides (chlordane, lindane, parathion).

Chlorinated water, chlorox, bleaches.

Sulfur dioxide, cedar-scented furniture polish, pine odors from knotty pine interiors and pine-scented household deodorants, bath oils, turpentine-containing paints.

In addition, many drugs contain chemicals, incuding aspirin, tranquilizers, sedatives and antibiotics.

Cosmetics nearly always contain chemicals, including toilet soaps, shampoos, hand lotions, antiseptic preparations, face powders, lipsticks, nail polish, mascara, hair sprays, perfumes, colognes, shaving lotions, hair dressings, scented toilet paper and douches.

Foods may be chemically contaminated in a number of different ways, including coloring added to hot dogs and to the rinds of fruits and vegetables (orange to make citrus fruit look more orange; red coloring to make apples look redder, etc.) Fruit and vegetables may also be waxed, or contaminated by insecticides or by wrappings derived from petrochemical sources.

Finally, tobacco pollutes the environment of many people.

Your level of chemical tolerance: If phosgene, chlorine and other poisonous gases are released, everyone who breathes them will be poisoned. Illness from such chemicals is called "toxicity." By contrast, indoor and outdoor pollution from chemicals including formaldehyde, insecticides, weed killers, diesel fumes and other industrial odors, may make some individuals sick; while others seem to remain well.

Whether or not you'll be made ill by exposure to chemicals appears to depend on several variables, including:

1. Your inherited tendency.
2. The load of chemicals you're exposed to.
3. Your load of other allergy troublemakers (foods, pollens, molds, etc.).
4. The integrity of your immune system (see, also, pages 9-10 and 163-166).

Managing chemical sensitivities: If you show symptoms from any chemicals, you're apt to develop sensitivity to other chemicals . . . especially if you're exposed to them in quantity over a prolonged period of time. *So one of the best ways to treat chemical sensitivity is to lighten your chemical load at home and at work.*

Since we're polluting our planet with automobile exhaust, industrial wastes, insecticides, weed killers, perfumes and other chemicals, keeping your chemical load low poses difficult problems. Yet, by learning about chemicals and by planning your life so as to avoid them, you'll increase your chances of remaining well.

Your understanding of chemical sensitivity will be made clearer if you understand the term, "outgassing." This term refers to the volatility of a material . . . its tendency to discharge molecules into the air.

As a rule, hard materials outgas less than soft materials. And natural substances outgas less than synthetics. Marble and stone are the least outgassing substances. And, of the man-made materials, ceramic tile is the least volatile. Soft plastics and polyurethane foam rank among the strongest outgassing substances. Other offenders include smokes, perfumes and sprays.

Here's a list of materials in your home which may cause problems:

Your Bedroom:
Foam rubber pillows or pillows made of other synthetic materials.

Mattresses covered with plastic and other synthetic material. Even cotton mattresses may be treated with fungicides and insecticides.

Sheets made of polyester.

Blankets . . . wool blankets may be treated with chemicals to make them less flammable or to keep moths away.

Pajamas & nightgowns may be made of polyester or other synthetics. (Use, instead, those made of cotton or silk.)

Floors . . . most floors today are covered with carpets which are made of chemicals. Moreover, carpet pads often are made of rubber or other outgassing materials. Some of the glues are even worse. Ideally, floors should be of ceramic tile, hardwood or stone with cotton scatter rugs. (Of the carpets, nylon with jute backing is best.)

Chairs & furniture. Many of these outgas, especially naughahyde, stuffed furniture containing foam rubber padding, or even cotton padding treated with insecticides.

154

Other chemical contaminants in your bedroom include perfumes and other cosmetics, hair sprays, tobacco smoke, synthetic curtains, floor waxes, television sets (put out an odor of phenol), and clothing.

Living room, family room and other rooms in your house:
Many of these rooms contain the same carpet as your bedroom. They also contain sofas, chairs and other materials that may outgas and cause trouble. Tobacco smoke is a common problem in many homes, either from the occupants or from visitors.

Kitchen:
Your kitchen is often loaded with outgassing substances, including a gas stove, soft vinyl flooring, soaps, detergents, insecticides and cleaning substances. Plastic dishes and Teflon® skillets may cause trouble in highly susceptible individuals.

Bathroom:
Your bathroom is often loaded with chemical odors, including cosmetics, soaps and deodorants. And even the chlorine odor from water causes trouble in some people. Plastic shower curtains may also offend.

Garage & Yard:
Gasoline and especially diesel odors cause problems in many people. This is especially true if the garage is connected to the house, and more especially if the garage has closed doors and lies under the house. Weed killers, bug killers and other chemicals stored in the garage may also cause trouble.

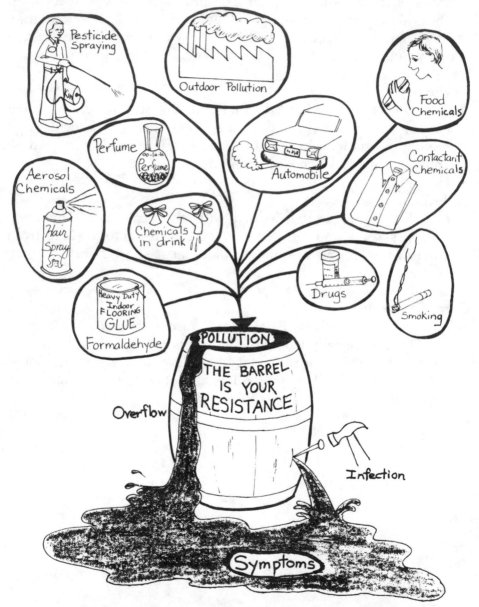

Adapted from William Rea M.D. Used with permission.

24

How Chemicals Make You Sick

You may be able to drive in traffic without experiencing symptoms; and chlorine and other chemicals in your drinking water may not bother you. You may also tolerate laundry detergents, furniture polishes, bathroom chemicals, perfumes and colognes. And you may tolerate foods containing coloring and additives or foods which are wrapped or stored in plastic.

You may also be able to go to a party or attend a conference in a room filled with tobacco smoke.

Yet, if you suffer from an immune-system disorder and your health problems are yeast connected, you're apt to be bothered by chemicals. And you may develop burning eyes, stuffy nose, itching, tingling, headache, muscle and joint pains, and all sorts of strange mental and nervous symptoms when you're exposed to outgassing chemicals.

Studies by Dr. William Rea[24] and others[25a,b] show that chemical exposure adversely affects many parts of the immune system. And the more chemicals you're exposed to, the greater the adverse effects.

If you're troubled by allergies and chemical exposures of any type, the "barrel concept" of Dr. Rea may help you understand how chemicals affect you.

Chemicals you're exposed to resemble pipes draining into a rain barrel. The barrel represents your resistance. If heavy chemical exposure continues, the barrel overflows and you develop symptoms. Also, infection often precipitates a "leak in your barrel," even when the barrel isn't full.

25
When Candida Is Treated, Your Chemical Sensitivity Will Often Improve

In September, 1982, 27-year old Mary Ann wrote:

"My general health has been reasonably good, although I've taken Keflex® and other antibiotics a couple of times a year for sore throat. Also, while on birth control pills several years ago, I was bothered by severe depression and irritability.

"Several months ago, while driving, I developed a strange sensation in my head and blacked out. –It was a terrifying experience and I feared for my life. Three weeks later I had a trance-like experience along with a funny taste in my mouth. Soon thereafter, my symptoms went wild. I developed strange sensations in my head off and on all day, with one or two black-outs a day, extreme fever, nausea, difficulty in breathing, sinus problems, heart irregularities and emotional instability. My headaches were severe.

"I consulted a neurologist who hospitalized me for a complete workup, including CAT scans and brain wave tests which were said to be 'just slightly irregular'. And because of questionable findings on the CAT scan, an arteriogram was carried out.

"Meanwhile, I had been put on Dilantin®. When the arteriogram showed no problem in my brain, my medicine was changed to phenobarbital.

"I was exhausted all the time and I felt awful trying to run a business and carry on as a wife and mother. My headaches persisted and I was so dopey I couldn't function well at all. My doctor and his nurse seemed to feel I was 'making much out of nothing' and wouldn't return my calls. So I found another doctor. By the way, the first doctor diagnosed me as epileptic and would not let me drive.

"The new neurologist said he couldn't fit me neatly into any category, such as epilepsy or brain tumor and that it was perhaps just 'nerves'. But to make sure, he would do another CAT scan, EEG, EKG and lumbar puncture. However, he told me to slowly wean myself off the phenobarbital which is where I am now. Yet my symptoms are recurring.

"Then last week I remembered developing an extreme reaction . . . dizziness, headaches, coughing . . . when we had cabinets built in the shop I was remodeling. This happened last March. The cabinets were built of pressed wood (containing formaldehyde) and I sat beside them daily. Also, I personalized gifts all day using enamel paints, paint thinners and turpentine. Moreover, the building I work in is poorly ventilated because my electric heat and air conditioning do not draw in outside air. The building is also very old and the back rooms are dusty. I also receive merchandise packed in straw which has been treated with formaldehyde.

"After reading recently about chemical sensitivity, I'm relieved to think that this might be my problem. Yet I'm desperate for help."

Because Mary Ann lived in another state and found it impossible to come to my office for a visit, after reviewing her history and because of her chemical sensitivity, I sent her personal physician information about yeast-connected illness. I suggested a therapeutic trial of nystatin, diet and nutritional supplements and changes in Mary Ann's work place so as to lessen chemical exposures. Six months later, in March, 1983, Mary Ann came in with the following report:

"I've improved to some degree, even though my physician decided not to prescribe nystatin. Yet, I'm still sensitive to many chemicals I come in contact with in the car and elsewhere."

After re-reviewing Mary Ann's history, I prescribed a therapeutic trial of nystatin, diet and nutritional supplements.
In a follow-up report in July, 1983, Mary Ann wrote,

"My improvement has been amazing . . . more than I expected. I've been on all-day car trips with no problems. The greatest thing that has happened is the nervousness, grouchiness and irritability that I thought was 'just me' has gone. The first two weeks on nystatin were terrible, but then I began to improve amazingly. My 4-year old daughter recently commented, 'Mommie, you don't fuss like you used to'.

"For a while I wasn't able to cheat on my diet without experiencing depression, but now I can eat anything although I still adhere to the diet most of the time.

"My monthly period is no longer a time I consider committing myself to a mental hospital. I feel great even then . . . and I certainly wasn't expecting this.

"I've never had so many compliments on how good I look . . . it all shows doesn't it? My husband lost 14 pounds on the diet and he feels beautiful, too.

"I have to admit now that I was very skeptical when I first came looking for help. Now I'm a real believer and it's such a wonderful relief to know I'm not just naturally an old grouch.

"I know now my problems began when I started taking birth control pills 13-years ago which contributed to my nervous breakdown. It's truly an answer to my prayers to find relief for so many of my physical and mental problems."

John Smith, M.D. (name changed), a 40-year old physician lived in the suburbs of a large city. John was bothered by many health problems, including severe chemical sensitivity. In searching for help he underwent many different tests and therapies, including hospitalization in an environmental unit. Yet, his chemical sensitivity continued.

Dr. Smith commented,

"I had to live like a hermit. I moved to a rural area, ate organically grown foods, drank spring water and avoided all petrochemicals and synthetic products, including those found in clothing and housing. Any break in my routine triggered symptoms.

"Then two years ago, I learned of the work of Dr. Truss and began taking nystatin and a low carbohydrate diet, plus nutritional supplements including garlic. Gradually my immune system improved and my chemical sensitivity lessened. More recently I've found that other anticandida therapies have helped, including inhaling amphotericin B powder and using the herb tea from the South American LaPacho tree.

"Although it's been a long struggle, I'm excited to report that I'm able to travel, eat in restaurants and I no longer have to follow my diet as closely as I once did. I've been able to rejoin the human race! Anticandida therapy has certainly played a major role in helping me and my immune system recover from severe chemical sensitivity."

The stories of Mary Ann and John clearly illustrate a number of important points that I've talked about in various parts of this book, including:

1. Each person with yeast-connected illness differs from every other person. Yet, common threads run through the histories of many patients.

2. Birth control pills (while tolerated by many women) have triggered severe and complex illnesses in many of my patients.

3. Antibiotics, especially "broad spectrum" drugs (while they save lives and relieve suffering) are a "two-edged sword." By encouraging yeast growth, their use often leads to other chronic health problems.

4. When the immune system is adversely affected, symptoms in-

volving every part of the body often develop. The endocrine, digestive and nervous systems are especially affected.

5. Intolerance to environmental chemicals is found in many patients with yeast-connected illness. Such chemical sensitivity usually lessens following anticandida therapy.

6. Although such therapy increases a person's tolerance for chemicals, reducing the chemical load remains a sound part of therapy.

7. Nystatin and diet rank at the top of the list of treatment measures used in helping individuals with yeast-connected health disorders. However, in my experience, other measures are important in strengthening the immune system and speeding recovery. Included especially are vitamins, minerals, garlic, linseed and primrose oils and sugar-free yogurt. For a more comprehensive discussion, see Section D.

8. Still other patients are helped by additional therapies, many of which are discussed in Section E of this book.

About Your Immune System And How It Protects You[†]

All around you are harmful substances that can "do you in" . . . bacteria, viruses and chemicals.

Yet, you survive. Here's why: You possess "the most stunning, effective protection the world has ever seen . . . your immune system." Like the army, navy, marines and airforce, your immune system is composed of a number of defenders with different capabilities.

These defenders hold harmful organisms in check and retard their growth. Occasionally, they even kill a few. *However, in the end, it is your body itself which must destroy the harmful organisms.* Your body must clean up the battlefield, seek out and destroy each germ. No matter where these germs hide, it is your body that must do the killing. Among your body's 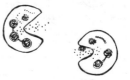 defenders are several types of white blood cells. And one group of these cells (called *granulocytes*) chase germs and gobble them up.

If you put these white blood cells in a small dish of salt water, they'll move around randomly in a tranquil manner. Yet, all you have to do is add one bacterium to the dish . . . just one . . . and the whole scene changes. The granulocytes, like a cat stalking its prey, creep relentlessly toward the bacterium. Then they attack. Later, they back off and let a different army of germ-fighting cells called *macrophages* take over.

Under the microscope you can see these different white blood cells

---

† Excerpted and adapted from *The Body is the Hero* by Ronald T. Glasser, M.D., Random House, 1976.

fighting for your life. You can actually see them grab bacteria and hold them while they empty their granules on them; you can see the microbes twist and turn and finally break apart.

The second part of your immune system . . . your *antibodies* . . . are special proteins circulating in your blood stream. A protein, as you may know, is made of linked-together *amino acids.* And they can be made to fit around almost any "foreign" structure. In so doing, they help you conquer your enemies.

How do the antibodies work? They clump microbes together and slow them down a bit, making it easier for granulocytes to eat them. They also unlock a series of physical events which lead to the microbes' death.

In addition to white blood cells and antibodies, the third and perhaps the most important part of your immune system is a group of nine separate proteins made in the liver called *"complement."* When activated, these complement components unite and help destroy the bacteria.

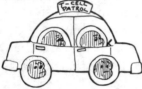

Among the other parts of your immune system are *lymphocytes.* These white blood cells patrol the body, making their rounds a hundred times a day. They are manufactured in the lymph nodes. The outer part of each lymph node is filled with "B" lymphocytes and the inner part with "T" cells or "T" lymphocytes. *These lymphocytes comprise the master mind of your immune system.* They'll attack bacteria, even ones you don't have antibodies against.

All parts of your immune system are needed to keep you healthy. In his book, *The Body is the Hero,* (see Reading List, page 275) Dr. Ronald J. Glasser commented,

> "To cure a disease, not just to treat it, you must help the body to do it itself. It is the body that is the hero, not science, not antibodies, not machines or new devices. It is the body making antibodies against the swallowed polio vaccine, not the iron lung, that cures polio. It is the body, not radiation or drugs, that must destroy cancer cells if the patient is to survive."

There is growing evidence that if you're troubled with allergies, chemical sensitivity, chronic and recurring infection, including candida, with symptoms which involve just about any and every part of

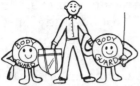

your body, it is your body which must be strengthened. And for your body to resist the harmful substances around it which are making you ill, your body's immune system must be on the job and functioning well.

Many different factors play a role in strengthening (or weakening) your body's immune system. These include:

1. The presence of excessive numbers of candida organisms in your intestinal tract and other parts of the body. And large numbers of candida organisms appear to put out a toxin which weaken your immune system.

2. Molds in your environment.

3. Chemicals you eat, breathe and touch.

4. Your nutritional status. A diet loaded with *sugar* interferes with the function of your granulocytes[6]. Similarly, a diet loaded with hardened fat, white flour, sugar, and other processed food lacks many essential nutrients your body needs to function properly.

These nutrients include essential amino acids (from proteins), complex carbohydrates (found in vegetables, fruits and whole grains), essential fatty acids (found in unprocessed vegetable oil), and a variety of vitamins and minerals.

Moreover, as pointed out by Roger Williams,[26] Ph.D. of the University of Texas, and Sidney Baker, M.D.[27a,b], head of the Gesell Institute in New Haven, Connecticut, *each person is biochemically unique.* And some individuals require much more of a particular vitamin . . . such as vitamin C or vitamin B-6 . . . than do others.

Minerals are still another story. And according to the late Henry Schroeder, M.D., Ph.D.[28] of Dartmouth College, *your mineral needs are even more important than your vitamin needs, since your body cannot make minerals.* You not only need the minerals found in large quantities in your body (such as magnesium and calcium), you also need many *trace minerals* including zinc, chromium and selenium.

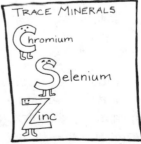

TRACE MINERALS

Chromium

Selenium

Zinc

These trace minerals are essential for taste, appetite, growth and for the proper functioning of your immune system and for many of the other metabolic and biochemical processes which keep your body strong and disease-free.

Studies by Pauling[29] and others indicate that vitamin C strengthens the immune system. Other studies show similar results. For example, in 1980, Anah and associates [30] told of a double-blind study on 41 Nigerian asthmatics who had noted increased asthmatic symptoms during the rainy season (suggesting mold sensitivity).

Twenty-two individuals were given 1000 mgs. of ascorbic acid (vitamin C) daily, while 19 other patients were treated with a placebo (dummy pill) for the 14-week duration of the rainy season. The group of patients who received no supplemental vitamin C experienced 35 asthmatic attacks, while the vitamin C group suffered only 9 such attacks. Subsequently, vitamin C was withheld from the individuals in group A and "the asthma attack rate increased remarkably."

Psychological factors are important. The late Dr. William Osler of Johns Hopkins pointed out that people who develop severe tuberculosis are often unhappy people. More recently, experiments in biofeedback show that you can speed up your heart or slow it down, or even regulate your blood pressure. And psychological factors may determine whether or not a person recovers from cancer.

A fascinating story about the role of psychological factors in curing a severe chronic illness can be found in Norman Cousins' book, *Anatomy of an Illness*.[31] Cousins, a former editor of the *Saturday Review of Literature,* developed a severe, crippling and supposedly incurable illness. Yet he got well. And he attributed his recovery to large doses of vitamin C, plus measures designed to make him laugh, along with a positive attitude and an intense desire to get well.

In his book, *The Body is the Hero*, Dr. Glasser commented,

> "The idea that an individual can control his immune system doesn't seem so far fetched anymore." And he suggested that we could use our minds to "will our white cells into a more efficient attack against infection."

Dr. Glasser continued,

> *"The task of the physician today is what it has always been, to help the body do what it has learned so well to do on its own during the unending struggle for survival . . . to heal itself.*

And if you suffer from yeast-connected health problems, your task is to learn as much as you can about the many things that play a role in making you sick, and do your best to cope with them. *After all, your body is the hero, and your body will recover if you'll give it a chance.*

27

Labelling Diseases Isn't The Way We Should Go†

In a paper some 10 years ago, E. Cheraskin,M.D., D.M.D.[22], then Chairman of the Department of Oral Medicine at the University of Alabama, said in effect,

> "We physicians are taught to diagnose, classify and label 'diseases'. And most of us feel if we can put a diagnostic label on each patient who comes to us, we've done our duty. Then we feel we can relax because our task becomes easy. All we have to do then is to go to our procedure book, medical library, Physicians Desk Reference® or computer and find the recommended treatment. Then we prescribe drugs, surgery or psychotherapy."

Cheraskin emphasized

> "There's a better way."

And in his numerous publications, including his book, *Predictive Medicine*[23], he pointed out that many disabling health disorders could be prevented by recognizing early signs and symptoms and helping patients make appropriate changes in their life styles and, more especially, in their diets.

In his recent book, *The Missing Diagnosis*[5], Dr. Orian Truss commented,

> "I would like to call attention once again to the pitfall inherent in dividing human illness into 'diseases'. The organs and systems of the body are so integrated, with each playing its specialized role in the maintenance of good health and efficient function, that to speak of disease of an individual organ is to suggest an autonomy that is underserved. If one organ

---

† Illustrations adapted from Sidney Baker, M.D., and used with permission.

167

malfunctions, it is likely that there will be repercussions in most other systems."

And recently Dr. Sidney Baker commented, saying in effect

> "Labelling diseases isn't the way we should go. And in working with people with the yeast problem, we need to take a new look at illness in terms of the differences between people. This is the important thing, rather than using so much of our time and energy trying to put labels on diseases, whether it be psoriasis, multiple sclerosis or Crohn's disease."

I agree. Although labelling disorders such as migraine, ulcerative colitis, asthma, the attention-deficit disorder, multiple sclerosis, or systemic lupus erythematosus serves a useful purpose, new scientific data suggest that many of these diseases are interrelated and result from environmental, nutritional, biochemical and other influences that affect the immune system. By recognizing these causes, and taking steps to alter them, physicians may be able to help many of their patients without resorting to hospitalization, surgery or drugs.

As physicians, we're taught to label diseases and divide them into separate and seemingly unrelated compartments. Some diseases are considered to be "mental" and to have mainly psychological causes, while others are categorized as being "physical."

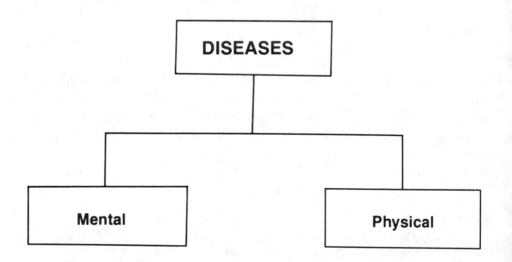

The mental diseases are usually divided into the following categories:

1. *Psychotic* ("crazy", disoriented, out of touch, paranoid). Treatment of such patients often includes custodial care.
2. *Neurotic* & nervous, ("can't cope," hypochondriacal). Psychological explanations are usually furnished (rejection, inadequate personality, sexual or religious worries, etc.).
3. *Childhood disorders.* Applied to those whose symptoms began early in life.
4. *Organic.* Caused by infection, trauma, poisoning or hardening of the arteries.

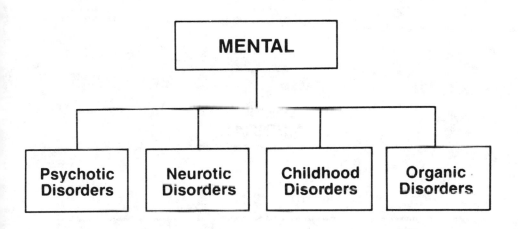

The physical diseases are also split up. Some are handled by medical doctors and others by surgeons.

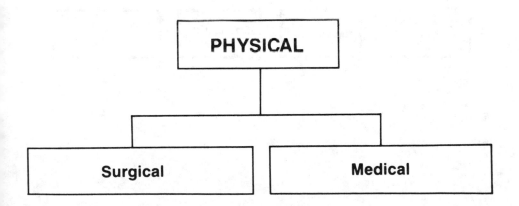

Then they are subdivided into organs or systems.

If you suffer from yeast-connected illness, you'll usually show symptoms involving your brain, your gastrointestinal tract and your reproductive organs. Yet you may also be bothered by symptoms in your bones and joints, your skin, your respiratory tract, urinary tract or other parts of your body.

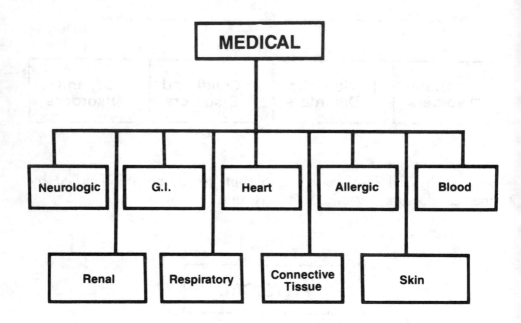

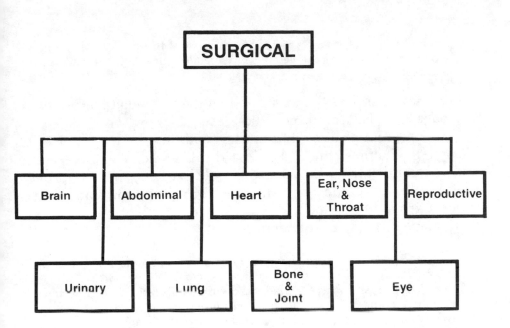

I'd like to acknowledge once again that the advances made by medical science during the past several decades are remarkable. Moreover, suffering is often relieved and health care costs are lessened by appropriate diagnostic and treatment procedures carried out by contemporary specialists and subspecialists. But there is "another side of the coin" as illustrated by the story of Carol.

For years, Carol had suffered from fatigue, headache and depression. She was also troubled by persistent and/or recurrent symptoms involving almost every part of her body.

Her nose was always stopped up and her throat was sore. And she coughed intermittently. Yet, allergy tests for inhalants showed no significant reactiions. Her menstrual periods were irregular and she often bled excessively. She also experienced repeated bouts of vaginitis and cystitis.

Carol was also bothered by bloating and other digestive complaints, including abdominal pain and constipation alternating with diarrhea. And she was rarely free of scaly skin rashes involving her hands and feet.

In talking about her health problems, Carol commented:

"During the past ten years my medical and hospital expenses have been more than $100,000. I've consulted internists, neurologists, dermatologists and psychiatrists. Every orifice of my body has been looked into and x-rays of every type have been made. My tonsils, uterus and one ovary have been removed and my bladder outlet has been dilated repeatedly."

I first saw Carol early in 1982 and on the Candida Questionnaire (see page 29), she scored over 300.

On a program of diet and nystatin (with intermittent courses of Nizoral®), vitamins, minerals, linseed oil, garlic, yogurt, exercise and immunotherapy with yeast and mold extracts, Carol improved remarkably. Love and understanding from her family and a lay-support group also helped.

In January, 1984, Carol commented:

"I've improved in every way and many of my symptoms have disappeared. However, on damp, muggy days I don't feel as 'with it' as I do on clear, crisp days. Tobacco smoke and perfume still stuff up my nose and give me a headache. Also, if I really cheat on my diet, I pay for it. But compared to the way I felt and looked two years ago, I'm a 'new woman'."

Patients like Carol are being helped by a small, but growing number of physicians all over the country. And as I pointed out in the Preface (see pages v-ix), "I sincerely feel that recognition and appropriate management of yeast-connected illness . . . will help physicians and their co-workers relieve much unnecessary suffering (and) . . . save patients, the government, business and industry (including the health insurance industry) billions of dollars."

28

Every Part Of Your Body Is Connected To Every Other Part

Obviously (although we often forget it), every part of your body is connected to every other part. Moreover, this interrelationship was clearly pointed out in the old spiritual song "Dry Bones" which went something like this. "Your foot bone is connected to your ankle bone and your ankle bone is connected to your knee bone" . . . and so on.

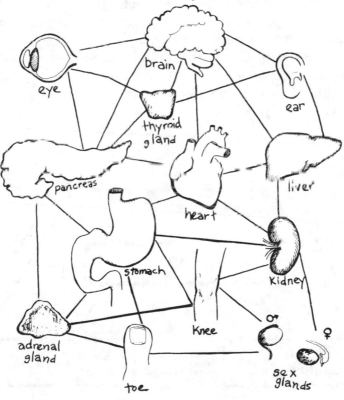

In my practice every day, I see many examples of these interrelationships. Here are two of them:

1. John, a 55-year-old business man, had been troubled with bloating and digestive problems for many years. He also was bothered by headache, buzzing in his ears and persistent athlete's foot. On the anti-candida treatment program, his symptoms subsided rapidly. Interestingly enough, John did not come to me as a patient originally; he only came along to give his wife emotional support. Then when he saw his wife improving, he said, "Can I go on the program, too?" He did, and he improved even more than his wife.

2. Louise, a 29-year-old school teacher was bothered by recurrent episodes of rhinitis and wheezing. Her problems were severe enough to require hospitalization. She also was troubled with premenstrual tension, fatigue, depression and menstrual irregularity. Her respiratory symptoms persisted even though she took allergy extracts for several years. Helping Louise hasn't been easy. Yet, after following a comprehensive program of management for a year, many of her health problems have improved.

Among the more important and recently recognized connections are those between the *immune system*, the *endocrine system* and the *brain*. *And since candida toxins affect each of these systems and one system affects the other, the yeast connection can cause all sorts of symptoms.* Here are examples:

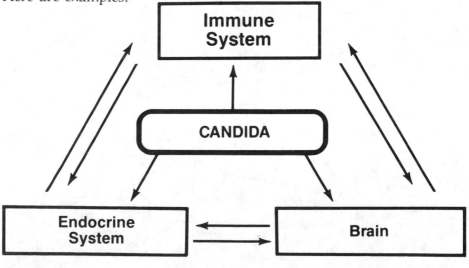

1. 33-year-old Barbara commented,

"Candida-related health problems made me tired, gave me headaches, irritability, menstrual problems and cystitis. And after the birth of my last baby, I lost all sexual feeling. Now, following three months of treatment with nystatin, diet, vitamins and minerals, it's just like it used to be. My husband and I are both grateful."

2. One of my patients, 27-year-old Anne commented,

"My nervous system wasn't working right. I was clumsy, uncoordinated and spaced out. My memory was terrible . . . worse than my 80-year-old grandmother's. At times my hands would be numb and would tingle. Following treatment, I feel better all over and my nervous system symptoms have disappeared."

3. Eleanor, a 25-year-old patient with headache, fatigue, constipation and recurrent vaginitis improved on diet and nystatin. However, she continued to be bothered by morning fatigue. And, at times, she would complain of feeling chilly. Thyroid and other tests were normal. However, her underarm thermometer reading in the mornings was usually 96° to 97°. Following thyroid supplementation, she improved more rapidly.

4. A gynecologist commented,

"I've seen several hundred young women with symptoms related to hormone dysfunction. These same patients were also experiencing candida related health problems. I've noted that by treating their yeast problems, premenstrual tension, menstrual cramps and other problems related to hormonal dysfunction improve . . . often dramatically."

In addition to the typical gynecological problems that have responded, many patients with other health problems, including arthritis, colitis, and other auto-immune disorders, have also improved. (See also pages 179-190.)

Section
D

Manifestations
of
yeast-connected
illness

Premenstrual
Syndrome

Vaginal
Problems

Menstrual
Difficulties

Small
Breasts

Skin
Problems

Painful
Intercourse

Pelvic
Pain

Headache

Fatigue

Depression

Irritability

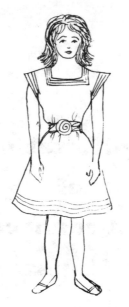

Infertility

29

Health Problems Of Women

Health problems of women are often yeast-connected. A young woman (I'll call her Sherry) went to her physician complaining of fatigue, menstrual irregularities and severe migraine headaches. Sherry was also worried about her poor breast development and remarked,

> "I dread going to the beach and putting on a bathing suit."

Following treatment with diet and nystatin, Sherry's headaches, fatigue, constipation, premenstrual tension and abdominal pain improved. And her breasts enlarged significantly.

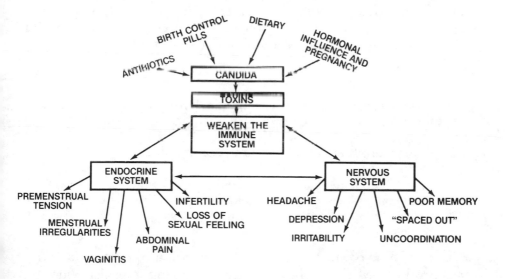

Recently, John Curlin, M.D., a Jackson, Tennessee gynecologist who has developed an interest in yeast-connected health problems commented,

> "Since entering practice, I've seen thousands of patients with symptoms related to hormone dysfunction. Their complaints have included pelvic pain, menstrual irregularities, PMS (premenstrual syndrome), infertility, nausea and vomiting of pregnancy, endometriosis, vaginitis, painful intercourse and absence of normal sexual interest and responsiveness.
>
> "Three years ago I learned of the observations of Joseph Miller[42] and Richard Mabray[43] who noted that women who experienced painful menstruation, premenstrual syndrome and other symptoms of hormone dysfunction often responded to tiny doses of progesterone. I began to use this method of therapy in patients in my own practice and found that many of them improved, often dramatically.
>
> "Then two years ago I learned about yeast related illness and began to use diet, nystatin and candida extracts in treating these patients. Although this program doesn't relieve all of the symptoms caused by hormone dysfunction, the response in most of my patients has been gratifying. In addition to the 'typical' gynecological problems that have responded, many patients with other health problems, including arthritis, colitis and other auto-immune disorders, have also improved."

Even though I was trained as a pediatrician, most of my new patients are adults . . . especially young women burdened with dozens of complaints involving especially their reproductive organs and nervous system. The response in many of these patients has been phenomenal . . . and exciting. Some of them give a history of marital discord and many have been divorced. A recent patient (I'll call her Laura) commented,

> "I was sexually unresponsive, depressed and irritable. I acted like a real bitch. No wonder my marriage failed."

And Mary, another recent patient, commented,

> "I was so hard to live with, my husband and I got a divorce. After getting off the pill and receiving anti-candida treatment, I'm married again . . . and to the same husband. And we're getting along just fine."

On June 25, 1983, just as this book was going to press, I talked to James Brodsky, M.D., a Chevy Chase, Maryland internist interested in yeast connected illness. Dr. Brodsky commented,

"I'm excited over the response of growing numbers of my patients to nystatin and diet."

Dr. Brodsky then told me about two of his female patients with "restless legs" whose symptoms vanished on anticandida therapy. Even more fascinating, he described the successful outcome of two patients who had been troubled with "the infertility problem." One patient had been trying to conceive for 7 months and the other for over 10 months. On diet and nystatin, one woman became pregnant in 30 days and the other in 60 days.†

I don't claim that an anti-candida treatment program will increase the brassiere size, banish infertility, cut the divorce rate in half or cure all the health problems of young women. Yet, it can work wonders in helping many women . . . and their spouses, too. What's more, women of all ages with chronic health disorders respond. Here are more detailed reports on some of my female patients:

I first saw Sara in 1951, a few hours after she was born. During the ensuing years, she came to see me dozens of times for routine checkups and for the treatment of colds and ear infections. During the 50's, she received many antibiotic drugs, including the tetracyclines. When Sara was 7 or 8, she began to sneeze and cough when she picked up a cat. About the same time, her mother commented,

"When Sara drinks chocolate milk she feels tired and develops dark circles under her eyes." On one occasion, she wheezed after playing in a wheat field.

Through her early and mid teen years, Sara enjoyed reasonably good health. Yet she often complained of feeling tired. She came in for a checkup at the age of 16 with the complaint of "falling asleep in study hall." She also was bothered by menstrual cramps, premenstrual tension and occasional episodes of vaginal yeast infection.

I didn't see Sara again as a patient until she was 27 when she came back to me saying,

"I'm wondering if my allergies have anything to do with my health problems."

---

† In September, 1983, a 34 year old patient from Memphis came in to see me with an infertility problem. She had been trying to have a baby for ten years. Four weeks after starting diet and nystatin, she became pregnant!

In going over her history, I found that she had continued to experience extreme fatigue accompanied by many other nervous symptoms. Sara commented,

> "I fall asleep anywhere and if I don't eat at frequent intervals I become weak. I'm also bothered by mood swings, frequent frontal headaches and severe menstrual cramps. And during the past 6 to 8 years, I've been treated repeatedly for vaginal yeast infections and cystitis."

Her records forwarded to me by her internist included two glucose tolerance tests. Both revealed elevations of her blood sugar level one-half hour after glucose was administered. On one occasion it went to 212 and on another it went to 221. Sugar also appeared in her urine. Then at the third and fourth hours, her blood sugar dropped rapidly; on one occasion it went to 41.

In talking further to Sara she said,

> "I feel dizzy on getting up and at times I feel 'real spaced out' like I'm not on this planet. My memory has been poor during recent years and at times I can't remember the names of people I know well. I feel uncoordinated, I stumble and drop things. My arms and legs ache."

Because of the complexity of her problems, I referred Sara to an endocrinologist for further study and treatment. She was hospitalized and, after a comprehensive work-up, her physician recorded this diagnosis in her chart: "Reactive hypoglycemia, symptomatic, with associated narcolepsy." Her treatment program included a high protein diet, supplemental vitamins, avoidance of food allergens, including wheat, chocolate and milk.

On this program, Sara improved; yet she continued to be troubled by severe vaginal yeast infections and bouts of fatigue and lethargy.

She came to see me again in the summer of 1980, saying,

> "I wonder if I need further allergy testing."

As I reviewed her history, I said,

> "Sara, since you last came to see me, I've learned of the work of Dr. Orian Truss of Birmingham who feels that *Candida albicans*, the common yeast germ which causes vaginitis, plays an important role in causing health problems similar to those you've experienced over the years."

I prescribed nystatin, a yeast free diet and nutritional supplements.

Although Sara has experienced a few ups and downs, she has improved remarkably. When I last saw her in January, 1983, she said,

"I feel great. No headaches, no spaced out feelings, lots of energy, only occasional mild premenstrual cramps. Life is full and exciting."

Was candida "the cause" of Sara's multiple and complex health problems? No. Many other factors were involved, including food and inhalant allergies, hormonal dysfunction and metabolic problems. But based on her response to anti-candida treatment, plus my experiences in hundreds of other patients . . . especially young women . . . I feel Sara's illnesses were due to a weakened immune system and that the anti-candida treatment program has played a major role in enabling her to regain her health.

Now I'd like to tell about Cindy who was born in 1963. Although I saw Cindy on one or two occasions during infancy and childhood, she was usually seen by one of my pediatric associates. Over the years, Cindy (like other members of her family), was troubled by allergies of all sorts, including rhinitis, otitis and bronchitis. However, Cindy's main complaints were more wide-spread. When she was 10, her physician commented,

"Cindy complains of headaches, abdominal pain . . . she aches everywhere!"

Cindy came in for a checkup at the age of 14 with the complaint of "not feeling well for a long time." Her symptoms included shortness of breath, substernal discomfort, headache, nervousness and anxiety. Although her mother had noted that milk and corn contributed to her symptoms, she never felt well. Treatment of spring and fall hayfever with allergy extracts and medication helped a little; yet she continued to experience multiple symptoms.

At the age of 15, Cindy came to me as an allergy patient. Her mother commented,

"Cindy has been through the mill. She's been seen by numerous doctors and although some of her treatments have helped, she never really feels good."

On a program of allergy testing and treatment with food and inhalant extracts, Cindy improved. Yet she continued to be a difficult and complex patient who experienced all sorts of ups and downs.

In an effort to obtain help, she consulted many other physicians, including gynecologists and urologists. She was hospitalized for study on several occasions. Because of severe menstrual cramps, she was placed on birth control pills and antibiotic drugs were prescribed for her bladder and respiratory infections.

In July, 1982, after an absence of three years, Cindy (age 19) came in with many of her same complaints. These included severe premenstrual tension, menstrual cramps and recurrent bladder infections (she had been treated with Keflex®), recurrent vaginitis and abdominal pain. I commented,

> "Cindy, I've learned a lot since I last saw you. And I feel most of your problems are yeast-related. Let's start over again and see if we can help you get well."

I sent Cindy to a gynecologist (who was interested in yeast-connected health problems) for a checkup. He prescribed a diet and nystatin. Cindy returned to my office in May, 1983 and commented,

> "I feel much better. Although I'm occasionally bothered by burning on urination, muscle aching and headache, I feel better than I've felt in years. Nystatin and diet have enabled me to conquer my unbearable menstrual cramps, fatigue and many of the other problems which had plagued me. Avoiding milk, corn, chocolate and other troublemaking foods helps. So do my allergy vaccines and nutritional supplements. *But the most important factor in helping me really feel better and look forward to college is my treatment with nystatin and diet.*"

Here's the story of a patient whose health problems began over 25 years before I first saw her on May 24, 1983. Margie was born in 1940 and came in complaining of recurrent vaginitis, abdominal pain, asthma and severe sensitivity to chemical fumes and tobacco. Other symptoms included sugar craving, headache, itching, muscle aches, numbness, tingling, depression, poor memory and fatigue. Here are excerpts from the letter she wrote me:

> "As a child I was sick all the time with a runny nose and cough. I had pneumonia several times. During my teen years, I moved to another state for six years and my health improved. Then when I moved back home, I again began coughing and had further bouts of pneumonia. After I went to work in a flower shop, I started having asthma attacks. My doctor sent me to an allergist who ran tests. I took shots and quit smoking and I got better.
>
> "Then after taking birth control pills for five years, I started having

vaginitis. I stopped the pill and my vaginitis cleared. But then I began having asthma at work from colognes, perfumes, soaps and cleaning products. I improved a little after being retested and started on shots for dust, pollens and tobacco. And my lungs were better until I painted the inside of my house. Finally, I had to quit work because I was sensitive to the perfumes the people I worked with were wearing.

"At some point, because of vaginitis, abdominal pain and persistent menstrual difficulties, I had a hysterectomy and bladder repair. Before surgery, I had so many bladder problems I was given all sorts of drugs including Terramycin®, Keflex® and Ceclor®.

"After taking these drugs, my vaginitis came back and has been one of my worst problems during the past three years. In August of last year, I had pneumonia which developed after I polished my floors using an odorous floor wax. I was treated with Keflex®, Erythromycin® and cortisone.

"My home doctor saw me in April of this year and said, 'I think yeast allergies are a big part of your problem.' So he put me on a yeast-free diet, nystatin, and sent me to see you. The nystatin caused 'die-off' reactions and my vaginitis is driving me crazy. So here I am."

Just as this book went to press, Margie wrote me and said,

"I've been on treatment for a month. I'm somewhat better. I'm really sticking to my diet for the first time. I can now tolerate the nystatin and it's helping. So are digestive enzymes and linseed oil. The congestion in my head and lungs is definitely better, but my vaginitis continues. But now that I know why I've been sick so much and so long, I believe I can get well."

Here's the story of a more recent patient, Linda, who came in with severe premenstrual syndrome (PMS). This young woman first came to see me on May 3, 1983 on referral from psychologist, Cheryl Robley, Ph.D.:

Linda complained of anxiety, fatigue and many other mental and nervous system symptoms. Here are excerpts from her medical history written in her own words:

"I've been married for 12 years, have two sons . . . ages 7 and 3 . . . and a very loving, understanding husband. I've been a happy person who never complained. I've loved my role as a wife, housewife and mother. Like everyone else, I'd occasionally be upset or moody, but this was never a real problem. Gradually, over the past few years, my moodiness increased to a point where, within minutes, it could change either way, from depression to anxiety and then back again. I could feel it coming on, but I had no control over it. *I found that mood swings were especially severe during the five or six days before my monthly period.*

"Increasingly, I began to have 'attacks' where I would get so upset I would clinch my fists, grit my teeth, wring my hands and tense every muscle in my body. I'd feel like screaming. I wouldn't be able to sit down or lie down. I would usually end up getting in the car and driving until I calmed down. I would feel as though I'm MAD. During these times I would feel completely irrational; I could not calm down or talk to anyone. Thoughts would race through my mind and become exaggerated.

"Even when I wasn't having attacks, I found I could not cope without getting upset with any situation, such as a washer or dryer going out or my husband forgetting to call me and tell me he'd be late in coming home after work.

"I resented my duties as a housewife, cleaning, washing, cooking, going shopping. At times, I didn't even want to get up off the couch and tuck my two children in bed . . . that's awful!

"Until the birth of my second son, the only symptoms I can remember were severe tension headaches and pains in my left shoulder blade and shoulder joint which developed after I sat at the telephone and typewriter for hours at a time. After my son was born in 1979, I developed bladder infections and had to take a lot of antibiotics. Soon afterward, I began to notice nausea, stomachache and occasional diarrhea.

"In the last few years, insomnia has taken over. I don't fight the bed, I just lie awake . . . sometimes for 3 hours or more. I cry at anything. I've gotten to the point of not feeling loved . . . not trusting my husband, not feeling secure. My self-confidence has begun to diminish.

"The episode that sent me to Dr. Robley was provoked by my husband not calling me to say he'd play cards one evening. He didn't come home until late. By that time, I was a 'raving maniac.' (*This was four days before my period was due to start.*) I tried to talk to him but ended up screaming insults. When I got no response, I started hitting him. It scared me so bad that I got in my car at 1 AM and drove around until 3 AM. I prayed out loud that God would give me an answer. I was tired of battling this thing. Finally, I called my gynecologist who referred me to the psychologist who sent me on to see you.

"I'm tired of feeling this way, I want to feel happy again and be able to cope day to day . . . enjoy life, my husband and my two boys.

"During the many years of our marriage, my husband and I have been through many emotional stresses, including job changes, financial problems and all sorts of other things. Yet I was able to cope until the last several years."

I put Linda on "the anti-candida program," including a yeast free diet and nystatin. At a recheck visit on May 24, 1983, Linda said,

"I'm better. However, the acid test will be this week, since my period is due to start in 7 days."

Linda came back again on June 20, 1983.

"I'm much better! For the first time in three years, my premenstrual period wasn't hell. I got through it without any blowups. Although I still have a little vaginal discharge and some of my old emotional symptoms pop up occasionally, I can deal with them."

A Special Word About PMS (Premenstrual Syndrome)

In a comprehensive article in the June, 1983 issue of *Hospital Practice*, Doctors Robert M. Rose and Judith M. Abplanalp of the University of Texas Medical Branch at Galveston commented,

> "This syndrome has become a popular scape-goat for behavioral aberrations ranging from malaise to murder . . . . Largely as a consequence of media attention (it has changed) over the past few years from a relatively obscure clinical entity to a household word."

What is PMS? It is a group of physical and psychological symptoms which occur or are accentuated during the week or so preceding menstruation, and are relieved when the period starts. Physical complaints often include painful or swollen breasts, bloating, abdominal pain, headache and backache. Even more striking are the mental and nervous system symptoms, including especially depression, anxiety, irritability and behavioral changes.

What causes PMS and how should it be treated? It depends on who you ask. British gynecologist Katharina Dalton feels that women with PMS suffer from a relative deficiency of progesterone during the week before menstruation. She has found that relief can often be obtained through the use of progesterone vaginal suppositories.†

Other physicians studying and treating PMS have emphasized the role of emotional factors; still others feel deficiencies of vitamins A and B-6, magnesium and other nutrients are at fault. Other viewpoints include prostaglandin excess, progesterone allergy and immune and endocrine system disorders related to *Candida albicans.*

C. Orian Truss, in his writings, has repeatedly emphasized the role of yeasts in causing health problems in women, including PMS.[51],[52] More recently, an number of gynecologists have confirmed Truss' observations and are successfully treating many of their PMS patients with an anti-candida program.

Gynecologist Richard Mabray of Victoria, Texas recently commented,

---

† A number of gynecologists I've talked to have confirmed Dr. Dalton's observations.

"A large percentage of phone calls and visits to gynecologists are related to vaginal yeast infections. At best, they're a nuisance to the patients; they're costly; they cause pain and often interfere with normal sexual relations. Of even greater importance is the effect of yeast toxins on the whole person. *I'm increasingly impressed with the role of candida in causing a whole host of health disorders in women, including depression, irritability and the premenstrual syndrome.*

"The most exciting thing I'm involved in now is a new association of PMS clinics in Texas, Arizona, Colorado and Utah. We'll be studying patients using clinical, psychological and laboratory studies and we'll put our findings on computers. It'll take a while to generate the data we need but we should have a lot to report in another year or two."

Gynecologist A. Stephens Orr of Atlanta had this to say,

Today, January, 1984, the first thing I think about when I see a patient with severe PMS syndrome is the association of this disorder with chronic candidiasis. I look for yeast-connected PMS, especially in women who give a history of receiving repeated antibiotics, feeling worse on damp days, chemical hypersensitivity, intolerance to birth control pills and recurrent vaginitis.

"In patients with such a history, I prescribe nystatin and a low carbohydrate diet. I'm very happy with the response, so are the patients, including some who have been referred by psychiatrists and psychologists. Candida isn't the only cause of PMS and some patients don't improve until they've been on treatment for 3 to 6 months. Nevertheless, anti-candida therapy is an important addition to successful PMS management."

My observations in my own patients resemble those of Doctors Truss, Mabray and Orr. Candida certainly isn't "the cause" of PMS. *Yet I feel that in the patient with the characteristic history suggesting yeast connected illness, a trial of anti-candida therapy is warranted.* I've observed that diet, nystatin and nutritional supplements, including primrose and linseed oils (which are rich in essential fatty acids), zinc and vitamins B-6 and E, often work dramatically in relieving PMS and a wide variety of other health problems of young women (see also pages 290-291). Included among these are recurrent vaginitis, pelvic pain, headache, fatigue, irritability, depression, infertility and other complaints related to poor hormone functioning (small breasts, lack of sexual interest and response, and painful intercourse).

Moreover, other health problems which do not involve the reproductive organs and other parts of the endocrine system may also improve, including rhinitis, bronchitis, arthritis, bursitis. Since "everything is connected to everything else," what helps a woman's reproductive organs and endocrine system helps every part of her body.

Why Yeast Connected Illness Occurs More In Women, Especially Young Women

Many women with yeast connected illness are tired, depressed and feel bad all over. They tend to complain of aches and pains in almost every part of their bodies. The typical young woman with these symptoms has consulted many different physicians, including gynecologists, internists, urologists, otolaryngologists and neurologists. And because their complaints continue and no apparent explanation is found, they may be told, "You'll just have to

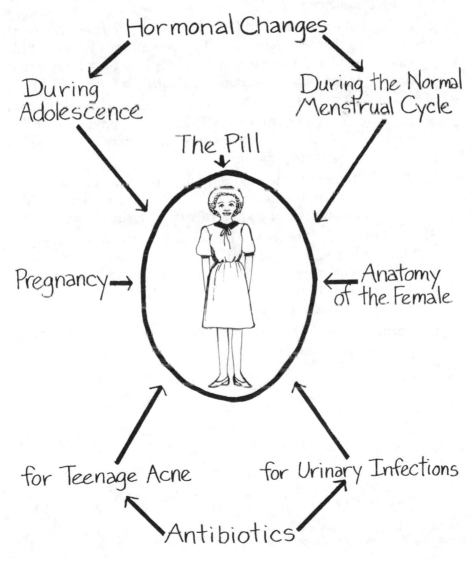

learn to live with these symptoms." If they continue to complain, their families, friends and physicians will usually label them as "hypochondriacs." And if their symptoms are severe and disabling, their physicians are apt to say, "I think you should discuss your problems with a psychiatrist."

Here's why females develop yeast connected health problems more often than males or children:

1. Hormonal changes associated with the normal menstrual cycle encourage yeast colonization†, as do hormonal changes during adolescence.

2. Hormonal imbalances and menstrual irregularities in women (including teenagers) are often treated with birth control pills. And "the pill" is a commonly used method of contraception. (Birth control pills encourage candida.)

3. Teenagers, especially girls, are concerned about their complexions. So they're more apt to consult a physician and be put on long-term tetracycline (or other antibiotics) as a part of an acne treatment program.

4. The anatomy of the female genitalia invites candida colonization. (The dark, warm recesses of the vagina provide an ideal home for families of candida microorganisms.)

5. The anatomy of the female bladder outlet (the urethra) is such that females experience urethritis, cystitis and other urinary tract problems more often than males. Broad spectrum antibiotics which promote yeast growth are often used in treating these disorders.

6. Hormonal and other changes associated with pregnancy encourage candida.

---

†Increased production of progesterone following ovulation results in changes in the vaginal membrane which promote the growth of candida.

Men, Too, Develop Yeast Connected Health Problems

Jim, a 36-year-old engineer, came to see me on February 23, 1982. His main complaint . . . . "athlete's foot for 20 years." For four years, Jim had also been troubled by other rashes involving especially his hands.

Jim commented,

> "I've been bothered with abdominal pain and sinus trouble off and on for many years. My energy supply is low and I experience a lot more fatigue than I feel is normal for a person my age. During the last 6 months, I frequently develop inappropriate drowsiness and trouble in concentrating. And at times I feel 'spaced out' and 'not with it'. These mental and nervous symptoms became worse when I went to work at an aluminum plant."

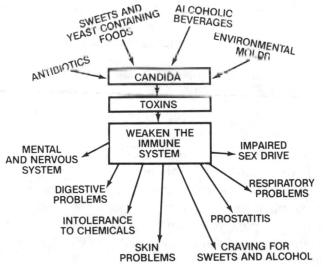

On examination, Jim showed what appeared to be a chronic fungus infection of his toenails plus a rash involving his fingers and hands. Following a blood test (the "liver panel"), I prescribed Nizoral® which Jim took for a year. In addition, I treated him with yeast and mold extracts which he took sublingually (under-the-tongue). He began to improve within a few weeks and at a checkup in February, 1983, Jim commented,

> "My rashes have disappeared and my nails are 95% well. My fatigue, nasal congestion, headaches and other symptoms are better, and my tolerance for environmental chemicals has improved."

Robert, a 31-year old refrigeration technician, came to see me on December 30, 1982 with severe hives and swelling. He was frightened and said,

> "I feel my throat is swelling and I have a lump in my stomach."

I gave Robert a shot of Adrenalin® which provided partial relief. In 30 minutes, I repeated the Adrenalin® injection.

In reviewing Robert's history, I found he had taken many antibiotics as a child. Then, while serving in the army, he developed a peculiar form of encephalitis or meningitis which was treated for several weeks with antibiotics, including tetracycline.

In 1979, Robert was again given a prolonged course of antibiotics because of "prostate infection." In 1981, he broke out in hives which persisted for a week. The rash returned in June, 1982 and recurred daily during the next 6 months. Medication included repeated Adrenalin® injections, Periactin® and Atarax®. Robert commented,

> "I've taken repeated courses of prednisone, and for the past two weeks I've been taking 30 to 60 mgs. a day. Yet my hives are worse."

In addition to his skin symptoms, Robert was troubled with nervousness, irritability, depression, joint pains and stiffness.

I put Robert on a yeast free, low carbohydrate diet, nystatin, nutritional supplements and taught his wife how to give injections of Adrenalin® and Susphrine®. Gradually, during the ensuing weeks, I was able to reduce his dose of prednisone.

Although during the past year Robert had his "ups and downs", his immune system has gradually recovered. At the time of his last visit, he commented,

"I haven't taken prednisone regularly for over 6 months. Yet, if I cheat on my diet or skip my medication, I'll develop a little itching."

George, a 36-year-old banker, came to see me on March 25, 1983. Here are excerpts from his letter :

"I've been bothered by sinus problems and sore throats all of my life. The severity varies and I've taken many antibiotics. For the past several months, I've felt light-headed and dizzy. I feel drained and 'zapped' most of the time and extremely anxious. In addition, I have spring and fall hayfever. I thought that my mental and nervous symptoms were caused by stress, but during a prolonged rainy period several weeks ago, I could tell I felt considerably worse. My sister who has been helped by diet and nystatin talked me into coming to see you."

Following allergy testing and a treatment program which included immunotherapy, diet, nystatin and nutritional supplements, George commented,

"All of my problems aren't solved, but I have more energy, feel less depressed and am enjoying life once more."

Paul, a 43-year-old factory worker wrote to me in February, 1983. Here are excerpts from his letter:

"As a child I was bothered by persistent colds and sinus congestion and during my early teens I took lots of antibiotics. Finally, when I was 16, my tonsils were removed and I got better. But by 18, I noticed that deodorants, colognes and perfumes gave me a headache and irritated my nose and throat.
"Soon afterward, I started working in a factory and my nose irritation, drainage, headaches and sore throats became worse. I took daily decongestants for several years and tried to stay away from perfumed soaps and deodorants.
"When I was 30, I bought an older home to remodel and began to work with panelling. About that time, I noticed more problems with my head, nose and throat. Then 4 or 5 years ago, my symptoms got worse and I began to have stomach trouble as well as head and throat trouble. A gastroenterologist made x-rays and used an instrument to look in my stomach. It showed only 'gastritis.'
"What really bothers me now is tobacco smoke at my work place. It sent me to the doctor three times in the last six months. Two minutes of smoke inhalation causes headache, tingling in my chest, dizziness, runny nose, burning eyes and mental confusion."

At the time of Paul's first visit on March 22, 1983, I put him on a comprehensive program of management, including nystatin, a yeast free, sugar free diet, extra vitamin C (2,000 to 3,000 milligrams a day) and nutritional supplements.

Paul steadily improved and at a followup visit on June 3, 1983, he said,

> "I'm much better. Now my bad days are as good as my good days were before I started treatment. My stomach no longer hurts; I don't need to take Tagamet® and my tolerance to tobacco and other chemicals has improved."

(Paul's wife, Betty, had been troubled with recurrent abdominal pain, respiratory problems and menstrual irregularity for years. Her stomach was x-rayed three times and a diagnosis of "nervous stomach and spastic colon" had been made. In May, 1982, her gynecologist prescribed nystatin and diet. Betty commented, "I feel better than I can remember feeling in a long time.")

In my practice, over ¾ of my patients with yeast connected health problems are women. *Yet, men, too, develop yeast connected health problems.* I particularly suspect such problems in men . . .

1. Who are troubled by food and inhalant allergies.
2. Who have been bothered by persistent "jock itch," athlete's foot, or fungous infection of the nails.
3. Who have taken repeated courses of antibiotics for acne, prostatitis, sinusitis or other infections.
4. Who consume lots of beer, breads and sweets.
5. Who crave alcohol.
6. Whose wives or children are bothered by yeast connected illness.
7. Who feel bad on damp days or on exposure to chemicals and/or tobacco.
8. Whose sex drive is impaired.
9. Who are troubled by fatigue, depression and other peculiar nervous system symptoms.
10. Who are bothered by recurrent digestive problems, including constipation, bloating, diarrhea and abdominal pain.

31

Health Problems Of Children

Although children differ from adults in many respects, many of the same factors which lead to candida colonization and a weakened immune system in adults also affect children. These include prolonged or repeated courses of antibiotic drugs and the consumption of diets with a high sugar and yeast content.

Yeast-connected illness should also be suspected in children whose parents have been bothered by similar problems. It is also more apt to occur in children who give a history of thrush and persistent diaper rashes.

In the summer of 1980, I was discussing the "American epidemic" of recurrent ear problems in children with another physician interested in yeast-connected illness. We both agreed that these problems seemed to be getting worse, rather than better. And in spite of polyethylene tubes and repeated or long-term antibiotics, ear problems were continuing to recur.

Since these drugs had encouraged candida and depressed the immune system in many of my adult patients, it seemed logical to prescribe nystatin for children who required an antibiotic for their ear infections. However, because I had limited my practice to allergy, I saw only an occasional child with ear problems. Accordingly, I had little opportunity to note the effectiveness of an anti-yeast program in children.

Then in January, 1982 I saw Rusty, a 5½ year old child with multiple health problems. He had been troubled with colic, recurrent colds, ear infections and hyperactivity during his first year of life. According to his mother,

"The doctor changed Rusty's formula several times. He was hyperac-

195

tive, even as an infant, but he was a smart baby who learned quickly.

"Rusty's constant colds continued and he averaged one ear infection a month. His developmental milestones were normal . . . sitting alone at 6 months, standing alone at 8 months, walking across the room at 11 months. His speech developed normally and by one year he could say 20 words. But then his progression seemed to cease. Around the age of 2 he became worse with increasing hyperactivity. Mild autistic symptoms began to appear and communication became an increasing problem; speech was broken and very fast."

Also, at age 2, the family moved into a new home which subsequently was found to be contaminated with formaldehyde. Rusty also ate lots of junk food. His recurrent ear infections continued and he always had dark circles under his eyes and a runny nose. Studies at a university medical center resulted in a diagnosis of "pervasive developmental disorder, with symptoms of autism."

At the time of his first visit to me, Rusty was put on the "cave man diet", a basic elimination diet† which avoided any and every food he ate more than once a week. After following this diet for a week, his mother reported,

"Rusty showed a dramatic improvement. He became more responsive and began to cooperate."

After challenging Rusty with mushrooms, his mother reported,

"Rusty became hyper, wild . . . aggressive, ill, crying, throwing things. Pupils dilated. Yeast caused a similar reaction."

Other foods, including wheat, corn and raisins also caused reactions . . . some of which were severe. For example, Rusty's mother reported,

"Thirty minutes after eating wheat, his pupils dilated and he stared into space more. Within a few hours he showed more autistic behavior."

The history of recurrent ear troubles treated with multiple antibiotic drugs, plus the sharp flareup in symptoms on challenge with yeast and mushrooms, made me feel that this child's problem was related, in part at least, to candida. Accordingly, as a part of his treatment program, Rusty was put on nystatin and a yeast and sugar

---

† *Tracking Down Hidden Food Allergy*, pages 25-38.

free diet. Within 2 or 3 months, Rusty improved to such an extent that three of his teachers wrote me a letter describing changes in Rusty's behavior and "dramatic improvement" in his readiness for learning. And on April 6, 1982, Rusty's mother sent me the following report:

> "Rusty continues to improve. He is now writing more of his ABC's and can write the alphabet in order down to H. He is using more language and putting words together, such as 'cook cookies', 'want to go'. His understanding of language is still improving, although speech is still fast. He is dressing himself and is awakening to the world!"

Between April, 1982 and December, 1983, Rusty's autistic behavior† and related developmental problems continued to improve. However, there were ups and downs. Exposure to chemical fumes caused a relapse; also, his family noted that larger doses of B vitamins, especially B-6, were essential for optimal functioning. Rusty still requires special education, yet his family is pleased with his progress.

---

† In December, 1983, I learned of another child with severe developmental problems, including autistic behavior, who improved on anti-candida therapy. The story of this child (Duffy Mayo) was described in the September 25, 1983 issue of the *Los Angeles Times* by Don Campbell.

On January 3, 1984, I called Duffy's physician, Dr. Alan Levin of San Francisco, to get more information. Here's what Dr. Levin told me: "During Duffy's first 18 months, his development was superior. Then because of recurrent ear infections, he received lots of antibiotics. Soon he began to slip backward and develop autistic-type behavior. He stopped talking, lost his vigor, and began withdrawing. He'd go from acting depressed and stuporous to 'climbing the walls'.

"When Duffy was about 3½, along with one of my colleagues, Phyllis Saifer, a Berkeley, California allergist and clinical ecologist, I began to study and treat Duffy using anti-allergy therapy. He began to improve. Subsequently, because of the history of antibiotic drugs, I prescribed nystatin and for a while he improved even more. Then I put him on the more potent anti-fungal drug, Nizoral®(ketoconazole) in a dose of one tablet a day. Later, another colleague, Dr. Cecil Bradley, increased the dose to two tablets and then to four tablets a day. Duffy improved dramatically and has maintained this improvement. Although he still shows some fine motor and comprehension problems, he's reading ahead of his milestones. I'm pleased and so is his family."

Was Duffy, like Charlie Swaart (see pages 229-230), actually drunk? According to Dr. Levin, no blood alcohol studies were carried out. Yet, before his anti-candida therapy, Duffy would stagger, giggle and break into silly laughs and act drunk. The research of Kazuo Iwata, M.D. of Japan shows that many candida species put out toxins. So regardless of whether it was alcohol or toxins affecting Duffy Mayo's nervous system, the trial of an anticandida treatment program helped.

Early in 1982, while I was working with Rusty, Truss' third article, "The Role of Candida Albicans in Human Illness," was published in the *Journal of Orthomolecular Psychiatry*. (This report was first presented at the Huxley Institute Symposium in September, 1981.) Although it dealt mainly with the role of *Candida albicans* in health problems in adults, Truss summarized,

> ". . . the categories of illness [in which he felt] the relationship to yeast is well established, those in which the evidence is strongly suggestive and those that I believe deserve careful study with respect to the possibility of such a relationship.
> "Infants and children with frequent infections and much antibiotic. Bowel disturbances, oral thursh, diaper rash, and respiratory allergy are common. Chronic irritability and hyperactivity, and even one case of stuttering, have been seen in children, many of whom carry the diagnosis of 'learning disabled'."

Truss also briefly discussed the manifestations of candidiasis in early adolescence,

> ". . . often with devastating effect on mood and on intellectual functions."

My interest in yeast-connected illness was further stimulated by the presentations at the Dallas Candida Conference on July 9, 10, 11, 1982. In the discussion period, several pediatricians told of their experiences in treating children with an anticandida program:

Dr. Aubrey Worrell:

> "Over the years, I've seen kids who are sick one week out of a month and each time they seem to require antibiotics. A year and a half ago, I began to use small doses of nystatin three times a day for 4 to 6 weeks. My patients seemed to do better. I think it works."

Dr. Morton Teich:

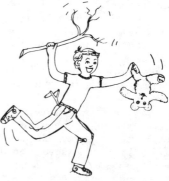

> "I've treated quite a number of hyperactive children and have done quite well with them, using the anticandida approach. One of our most significant findings in studying hyperactive patients was the history of sugar craving. This relationship is so striking that I've come to feel if a patient doesn't have some form of sugar and yeast craving, I tend to question the diagnosis."

Dr. Francis Waickman:

"Sixty percent of the illnesses which take children to doctors are viral. Yet, many of these viral illnesses are treated with antibiotics. In my opinion, stopping the overuse of antibiotic drugs in children is the number one way to lessen candida colonization. Most children with recurrent infections receive excessive amounts of sugar. And cutting down on sugar is the next most important thing physicians can do. I've had better results by paying attention to these factors than by giving nystatin."

Another pediatrician commented,

"Until recently, I had not developed a clear and consistent policy in dealing with this problem. But I'm now tending more and more to put my regular pediatric patients (who are given ampicillin or other broad-spectrum drugs for treatment of otitis media) on prophylactic nystatin. However, I feel that curbing the use of antibiotics is really the key."

In my general pediatric and allergy practice during the past 10 years, I've found that sugar is the *number one cause* of hyperactivity. Accordingly, the observations of Rusty's mother, along with those of the physicians at the Dallas Candida Conference, turned a light on in my "computer." And I easily recalled dozens of hyperactive children I'd seen whose mothers commented,

"Johnny's addicted to sugar. He'll cheat, lie or steal to get it. I have to watch him like a hawk."

I began to ask myself, *"Is it possible that my sugar-craving children who show hyperactive behavior when they eat sweets are developing these nervous system symptoms because sugar feeds their candida? And is this the answer rather than sugar allergy?"*

Perhaps it is, yet I realize candida isn't the whole story. Here's why: Several years ago, I carried out a clinical study on 10 of my hyperactive patients whose parents had reported,

"When my child eats sugar, he becomes hyperactive."

Here's what I did.

I bought 50 pounds of cane sugar and 50 pounds of beet sugar. I gave a 2-pound sack of both types of sugar to the parents of each of these hyperactive youngsters. And I outlined a special plan for giving them the sugar.

I won't review this study in detail. However, I was fascinated to find that *some children reacted to cane sugar who did not react to beet sugar, and some reacted to beet who did not react to cane. Some reacted to both sugars and some reacted to neither.* I've also observed on many occasions that foods containing corn sugar cause reactions in some patients. Yet, such patients may be able to take equivalent amounts of carbohydrates from other sources, including cane and beet. Also, many patients who react to cane, corn and beet may be able to take honey or maple syrup.

My brief study, along with my clinical observations, confirmed the findings of pioneer food allergist, Theron Randolph[32] of Chicago who, many years ago, noted that *sensitivity to sugar depends, in part at least, on the botanical source of the sugar. Accordingly, I feel that some sugar reactions are allergic or allergic-like, even though the mechanisms causing these reactions remain obscure.*

But now that I've become aware of candida-related illness, I feel some hyperactive children, especially those who have taken repeated courses of antibiotics, react to sugar because the sugar triggers candida.

During the past year, I've seen additional children in whom candida appeared to be a major thread in the "web" of their health problems. And I feel I now possess sufficient clinical evidence to change the way I treat children with ear infections, urinary tract infections, hyperactivity, behavior and learning problems and acne.

More specifically, when I treat a respiratory or urinary tract infection with amoxicillin, Ceclor,® Septra,® Bactrim,® Keflex,® or other broad-spectrum antibiotic drugs, I also prescribe nystatin during the time the child is receiving the drug. And if the child has taken antibiotics repeatedly over a prolonged period of time, I feel more prolonged courses of nystatin are indicated. In addition, I recommend a diet which eliminates yeast and refined carbohydrates, especially sugar and corn syrup.

In treating bacterial respiratory infections in children, I prefer penicillin V or penicillin G. Here's why: These drugs help mainly in eradicating the families of bacteria which cause respiratory tract infection and they do not wipe out the normal bacteria found in the intestinal tract. By contrast, the broad-spectrum drugs just referred to not only eradicate the harmful germs causing respiratory tract infections, they also wipe out many of the friendly germs found in the intestinal tract. And when these friendly germs are knocked out, *Candida albicans* moves in. (See, also, pages 10, 11.)

In treating urinary tract infections in children, I prefer Furadantin® or Macrodantin® since these drugs are usually effective and are less apt to encourage the growth of candida.

According to Dennis B. Worthen,[33] Ph.D., Chief, Information Services of Norwich Eaton Pharmaceuticals, Inc.,

" . . . Nitrofurantoin drugs, Furadantin® and Macrodantin®, have less effect on intestinal flora than do systemic antibiotics such as ampicillin, tetracycline, Bactrim® and Septra®. Since nitrofurantoin is effective only in urinary tract infections, concentrations in the gastrointestinal tract are not sufficiently high to significantly alter the normal flora. Consequently, the problems that would normally occur due to an altered flora/fauna balance are not normally observed."

In my experience, the causes of hyperactivity resemble a jigsaw puzzle. And to help the hyperactive child, many pieces need to be put into place, including attention to food allergies, nutritional needs, avoidance of lead and other toxic metals, appropriate light, good teaching, and so on. *However, if a hyperactive, learning disabled child gives a history of recurrent ear and other infections, and if his hyperactive behavior is triggered by sugar, I feel the anticandida program should be a part of his overall management.*

Here are further clinical reports indicating that the yeast connection plays a role in causing health problems in children, including ear problems and related behavior and learning problems:

In his book, *The Missing Diagnosis*,[52] Truss in his chapter on "Infants and Children," comments,

"The problem of chronic candidiasis in infants and children is especially important, not alone as it relates to their health at this period of their lives, but also as it may relate to problems with yeast later in life."

Truss points out that antibiotics are frequently given to children and that . . .

"after the use of antibiotic has been discontinued, the previous state of health may not return . . . Restlessness, discontent and irritability often accompany 'the runny nose'."

He also discusses other health problems in children, including learning disabilities and depression. He said,

"At any age, but particularly in young children experiencing difficulty

201

with school, this condition (meaning candidiasis) is one worth considering."

In March, 1983, Allan Lieberman, M.D., a South Carolina pediatrician, wrote me and said, in effect,

> "I treat almost every patient I see, including children with hyperactivity, behavior and learning problems, using a therapeutic trial of the anticandida program. The dramatic results I've obtained in so many encourage me to continue this approach. I've found that young children with recurrent respiratory and ear infections seem to really benefit. So do children, especially teenagers, with chronic depression."

About the same time, obstetrician and gynecologist, John Curlin, had this to say:

> "My 13-year-old daughter is quite an advanced and well coordinated gymnast. However, since infancy, she had shown periods of moodiness, depression and fatigue. And during the past year or so, she has noticed periodic changes in her ability to concentrate and coordinate her movements.
>
> "During the past year, we've learned that she *does extremely well if she maintains her diet and nystatin therapy.* If she does not, her moodiness and marked fatigue will return. And, interestingly, she'll show a lack of physical coordination in her gymnastics.
>
> "My 15-year-old son has been on a program of immunotherapy for inhalant allergies for over a year. Yet, he, too, has improved significantly by following his diet and taking nystatin.
>
> "Our youngest son, now 14 months of age, was fed only breast milk during his first six months of life and continued on breast milk plus other foods until the age of one year. Nevertheless, he was constantly irritable and suffered from a chronic rhinitis which would flare up without known causative factors.
>
> "*Almost within 24 hours after I began giving him small doses of nystatin powder, his rhinitis cleared and he showed a noticeable change in personality. His irritability subsided and he became much more pleasant.*
>
> "This is so impressive that family members can recognize when his daily doses of nystatin have been forgotten by the sudden changes in his behavior. Then when he receives his nystatin, he settles down."

Dr. Curlin's comments about his young son led me to speculate about some of the hundreds of crabby, irritable and colicky infants I've seen. Many of these babies experienced persistent abdominal pain and discomfort, regardless of formula changes or other treatment measures I prescribed. Moreover, I've seen many colicky or crabby infants who were totally breast fed.

202

Would a therapeutic trial of nystatin be appropriate for such infants? And would it be safe?

Again my answer is "Yes."

Abdominal discomfort and other digestive symptoms occur so commonly in adults with candida connected health problems it seems reasonable to anticipate that similar abdominal symptoms also trouble infants. Candida related colic† should especially be suspected in infants who have been troubled by persistent diaper rashes, and/or thrush, or whose mothers have experienced candida related health problems.

Ear Problems In Children . . . Isn't There A Better Answer?

In my opinion which is shared by thousands of physicians and untold numbers of parents, recurrent ear problems in infants and young children are one of the most perplexing dilemmas of the 1980's. One mother commented,

> "My two sons and just about all of my friends' children have had ear tubes. Isn't there a better answer?"

At a meeting of the Society for Clinical Ecology and Environmental Medicine, held concurrently with the annual meeting of the American Academy of Pediatrics (New York, October 24, 1982), Dr. George Shambaugh, Professor Emeritus of Otolaryngology at Northwestern University and a former President of the American Academy of Otolaryngology, gave an address entitled,

> "Serous Otitis: Are Tubes the Answer?"

In this address, Dr. Shambaugh commented,
"Serous otitis . . . *is the largest single cause of hearing loss in children.* And the operation of inserting a ventilating tube through the tympanic membrane (ear drum) to restore hearing has become the most frequent hospital surgical procedure with anesthesia today.

> "Removal of enlarged adenoids and tonsils in children, most of them with OME (otitis media with effusion) and with tube insertion, is the se-

---

† Obviously, candida isn't "the cause" of colic in all babies. If you need further suggestions for coping with an uncomfortable, unhappy baby, get a copy of Sandy Jones' new book, "Crying Baby, Sleepless Nights" (See *Reading List*, page, 278.)

cond most frequent operation. Together, these operations, along with treatment of acute otitis media in children, is estimated by Dr. Charles D. Bluestone of Pittsburgh (in an article in the *New England Journal of Medicine*) to cost two billion dollars a year. The estimated cost of one operation for adenoidectomy and tube insertion . . . for the anesthesia, operating room, surgical fee, two nights in the hospital . . . is $1,000 or more. I think mostly more."

In his continuing discussion, Dr. Shambaugh said, in effect,

"There's no question of the usefulness of ventilating tubes for OME to equalize the air pressure on both sides of the tympanic membrane, thus allowing the fluid to resolve or to be expelled by ciliary action to the eustachian tube.
"Yet, tubes alone aren't the answer for parents who are struggling to cope . . . often unsuccessfully . . . with the management of recurrent ear problems in their children. Neither are they an answer for their pediatricians, family physicians and otolaryngologists who are trying to help them."

Dr. Shambaugh urged pediatricians, otolaryngologists, allergists, clinical ecologists and other physicians to take a look at the allergic aspects of ear problems in children. And he commented,

"Although allergies in children are often hard to identify by the usual allergy scratch tests, I've found that a program of allergic management with attention to hidden or delayed-in-onset food allergy helps me manage recurrent ear problems in children. Moreover, my results with allergy management are far better than those obtained by putting children on prolonged courses of antibiotics and relying on tubes to clear up the condition."

Are Recurrent Ear Problems in Children Related to Candida?: I don't know. Yet, based on my experiences in treating hundreds of adults who developed yeast connected illness following prolonged or repeated courses of antibiotic drugs, such a relationship seems possible or even probable. Moreover, my own experiences in using nystatin and a special diet in a limited number of children with recurrent ear problems make me feel that an anticandida treatment program in these children is appropriate.

Here's a report on Wesley, a 4-year-old youngster I saw for a follow-up visit a few days before I finished the manuscript for this book and sent it to the publisher:

Wesley was born May 4, 1979 and had been seen regularly by his pediatricians. Here are items I excerpted from the medical record which was sent to me:

Treated for thrush and monilia diaper rash with oral Mycotatin® and Mycostatin Cream® to his diaper area at the age of 2 months. At 2½ months, thrush was still bothering him and gentian violet was prescribed.

At age 3 months, still having thrush; gentian violet treatment again prescribed. Ear infection noted at age 5 months, antibiotics prescribed. Began to have recurrent ear problems which responded poorly to antibiotics which he received on many occasions between the ages of 6 and 13 months.

Beginning June 1, 1980, more antibiotics were prescribed, including Pediazole®. Noted to be crying and irritable, was changed to Cyclopen® on June 9th. On June 17th, put on Ceclor® because of "persistent otitis media."

On July 1, 1980, Ceclor® was continued and on July 12 ears were noted to be 'finally looking better'. Put on Gantrisin® "suppression" . . . two 1-pint bottles prescribed, to be given 1 teaspoon twice daily.

On September 11, 1980 . . . irritable, picking at ears. Ears dull but not infected. Put on Septra®, 1 teaspoon twice daily.

January 31, 1981 . . . bilateral otitis. Amoxicillin prescribed.

February 14, 1981 . . . put on Cyclopen® for 10 days.

March 11, 1981 . . . In for checkup because of earache and hyperactivity. The child's mother commented,

> "Wesley periodically goes stark raving mad . . . wild . . . climbing the walls . . . chocolate and corn seem to provoke these symptoms. Chemicals, including colognes and after shave lotions do the same."

Cyclopen® prescribed for otitis. Mother phoned that Cyclopen® made his hyperactivity worse. Medication changed to Septra.®

April 4, 1981 . . . ears noted to be clear.

May 18, 1981 . . . respiratory infection, ears dull and red. Amoxicillin prescribed.

July 5, 1981 . . . viral infection, "ears look good without evidence of infection."

August 25, 1981 . . . in for checkup because of hyperactivity.

> "Having temper tantrums, beats his head and carries on for at least an hour. Bites his sister. Nothing seems to help. Attacks not brought on by frustration or being upset. Sleeps poorly, mother worn out."

Because of sleep problems, hyperactivity and prolonged 'fits' . . .
much worse than routine temper tantrums, referred to a clinical
psychologist.

December 28, 1981 . . . In with fever of 104° to 105°. Ears 'sharp
and clear'. Exudative pharyngitis. White blood count 20,800. Treatment . . . bicillin.

February 11, 1982 . . . left otitis media, given amoxicillin.

February 23, 1982 . . . ears still dull, 10 more days of amoxicillin
prescribed.

March 20, 1982 . . . otitis media, amoxicillin prescribed.

April 9, 1982 . . . ears clear.

August 17, 1982 . . . age 3 years, 3 months. Referred to me for consultation. Review of history showed that Wesley reacted to sweets of
any kind. Corn said to be a major troublemaker. The child also experienced episodes characterized by nasal congestion, swelling of the
mouth and bags under his eyes associated with hyperactivity. Anti-
yeast program prescribed, including yeast free, sugar free diet and
nystatin. Supplemental nutrients also prescribed, including linseed
oil and vitamins.

September 17, 1982 . . . much, much better. 'Like an entirely different child.' Challenged with 'junk food' . . . caused hyperactivity
and irritability.

October 15, 1982 . . . doing well. Sugar in any amount triggers
symptoms. So do apples. Nystatin being continued.

April 1, 1983 . . . in for recheck. Has been continued on diet and
nystatin, but taking only small 'dots' of nystatin two or three times a
day. Symptoms still recur on eating sweets.

Recommendations: Tighten up on diet. Give 1/16 teaspoon of
nystatin four times a day.

Follow up visit, May 1, 1983 . . . Comments by mother:

> "Wesley has had a great month as far as his hyperactivity is concerned.
> He's been on the nystatin in full force and a sugar free, yeast free diet. We
> only had one outbreak of the hyperactivity . . . this past Sunday . . . at a
> wedding anniversary celebration. He got some cake and punch. That night
> he was in terrible shape."

In her notes Wesley's mother commented,

> "I'm very sure that nystatin helps. Taking it on a regular basis four times
> a day has made a real difference as compared to taking it now and then.

We've had a great month. Wesley is so much better. He sits down and looks at books, he can be taken places without tearing the place apart. He's very cooperative and things are running so smoothly. As I said before, I really believe in the nystatin."

In his book, "The Missing Diagnosis,[52] Truss describes in detail

"a 16-month-old baby boy (who) was seen because of almost constant health problems that began at 2½ months of age."

At that age, because of cough and fever, the child received an antibiotic (Erythromycin®). One week later, Keflex® was prescribed. Although the child temporarily improved, he was seen at least once a month with recurrent respiratory problems, including ear infections. At 10 months, tubes were put in both ears. Health problems, including recurrent otitis, constant irritability and difficulty sleeping continued.

At the time of his first visit with Truss, the child was given a prescription for oral nystatin, 200,000 units four times a day as a liquid suspension. After one week of nystatin his mother reported he

"feels excellent — running around, clapping his hands. Just feels better all over."

After three weeks of nystatin, the medication was discontinued and the child's symptoms returned. Nystatin was again prescribed and continued for four months. The child remained well through the entire ensuing winter.

In commenting on this child, Truss noted,

"In my opinion, this is not an isolated problem. In fact, it probably is very common. Antibiotics save countless lives, but as with most forms of medical treatment some individuals are left with residual problems related to their use. . .

Perhaps the single most fascinating potentially important aspect of this case was the abrupt cessation of the ear infections. This suggests that *Candida albicans* was actually causing this problem and makes one wonder about the possible relationship of this yeast to what seems almost a national epidemic of otitis and tubes in the ears."

The response of Rusty, Wesley and other of my pediatric patients, along with the reports from other physicians, including Doctors Teich, Curlin and Truss, make me feel that *it is urgent for pediatricians, family practitioners, otolaryngologists and other physicians to*

207

know about "the yeast connection." Moreover, I hope these anecdotal reports will stimulate physicians, both in practice and in the academic centers, to carry out studies to document the relationship of candida to a wide variety of health problems which are troubling children and perplexing parents and physicians.

For example, one group of young children with ear problems could be given "the routine treatment"; a second group could be put on a special diet and 1/16 to 1/8 teaspoon of nystatin four times a day.

Candida isn't "the cause" of recurrent ear disorders. And like all health problems, such disorders are related to many different factors which combine to lessen the child's resistance. Yet, if the response of the children given nystatin and a special diet resembled that shown by Rusty or Wesley, much suffering and expense could be avoided.

Suggestions for Managing the Infant and Young Child with Persistent or Recurring Respiratory Disorders, Including Ear Problems:

1. Milk-Free, Chocolate/Cola-Free, Corn-Free, Sugar-Free, Citrus-Free, Egg-Free, Yeast-Free Diet.

Pediatricians and allergists continue to argue about food allergy and its incidence in infants and young children. Yet, many observers, [34a,b,c,d,e,f,g,h,i] including Deamer, Gerrard and Speer, feel that hidden or delayed-in-onset food allergy, especially cow's milk allergy, is a common cause of health problems in children. And they commented recently, "Far too many children have tubes put in their ears before allergy is even considered."

They also pointed out that "milk allergy is difficult to diagnose by the usual immunologic tests, including skin tests and RAST tests. Ogle and Bullock[35] made similar observations and urged physicians to use elimination diets in working with their young patients.

And in a study of 1000 patients with food allergy, Speer[36] found that milk, chocolate/cola, corn, citrus and egg were at the top of his list of "most common food allergens." Milk allergy was especially common in children under two.

Other observers[37a,B] have described the relationship of cow's milk to persistent rhinitis and other health problems in children. The Price-Pottenger Foundation[38] has also documented the relationship of cow's milk, especially heat treated cow's milk, to respiratory problems in kittens.

And the studies of Cheraskin and Ringsdorf[19] suggest that sugar and other refined carbohydrates lessen the ability of a person's phagocytes (germ eating white blood cells) to gobble up attacking germs.

So it seems possible that traditional sugar or corn syrup-containing cow's milk formulas in infants may play a role in causing health problems.

Putting all of these factors together, I've devised a feeding program for my infant patients with persistent or recurrent rhinitis and otitis. In addition, I suggest that foods be rotated to the extent possible to lessen the chances of other food allergies developing. (See, also, pages 129, 130.) Admittedly, this diet won't help every infant, and some 25% of milk-sensitive babies develop soy allergy. So Nutramigen® or goat's milk or other breast milk substitutes must be sought if human breast milk isn't available.

Here are the ingredients of this diet:

a. A special carbohydrate-free soy formula, RCF (Ross Laboratories). This formula is available in 13-ounce cans at most pharmacies, and contains a balanced amount of protein, fat, vitamins and minerals.

b. Carbohydrates are obtained from fruits, vegetables and whole grain cereals rather than from corn syrup or cane sugar. (A baby who takes a can of RCF per day needs 45 to 60 grams of carbohydrate.)

Sugar-Free Baby Food	Amount	Carbohydrate Content
Sweet potato	4¾ oz. (1 jar)	21 grams
Spinach	4¾ oz. (1 jar)	8 grams
Squash	4½ oz. (1 jar)	7 grams
Carrots	4½ oz. (1 jar)	7 grams
Beets	4½ oz. (1 jar)	7 grams
Peas, green	4½ oz. (1 jar)	8 grams
Pears	4½ oz. (1 jar)	14 grams
Applesauce	4½ oz. (1 jar)	15 grams
Fresh banana	½ small	11 grams
Apple-grape juice	4 oz.	16 grams
Apple juice	4 oz.	15 grams
Apple-plum	4 oz.	18 grams
Orange-apple	4 oz.	16 grams

Sugar-Free Baby Food	Amount	Carbohydrate Content
Rice baby cereal	6 Tbs.	11 grams
Oatmeal baby cereal	6 Tbs.	10 grams
Barley baby cereal	6 Tbs.	10 grams

Example: 1 jar of sweet potatoes, 1 jar of applesauce, 1 jar of pears, and 6 Tbs. of oatmeal cereal contains 60 grams of carbohydrate. Equivalent amounts of home-prepared food may also be used. Here are representative foods and their carbohydrate contents:

Baked potato	2½" diameter	21 grams
Black-eyed peas	½ cup	18 grams
Cream of wheat	½ cup	14 grams
Rice cake	1 cake	7 grams

I also recommend the following treatment measures:

1. Nystatin, 100,000 to 300,000 units (1 to 4 ml) four times a day for two to three months or longer (nystatin oral suspension — Squibb or Lederle), or nystatin powder, 1/32 to 1/8 teaspoon four times a day. (Nystatin powder can be obtained by any pharmacist from the American Cyanamid Company. See, also, page 44.)

2. Clean up the chemicals in the child's environment, including tobacco smoke, perfume, formaldehyde, floor waxes, bathroom cleaners and laundry detergents (see pages 152-155.) These substances irritate the lining of the child's nose and throat and adversely affect the immune system and make the child more susceptible to infections and allergies. Other environmental control measures should also be instituted so as to lessen exposure to house dust, molds and animal danders.

3. Additional vitamin C, 100 to 250 milligrams three or four times a day. Recent research, reported in the Abstract Section of the "Journal of Allergy and Clinical Immunology,[30] suggest that larger than usual doses of vitamin C may strengthen the immune system in allergic individuals. (See page 166 for a summary of the findings of this study.)

If a child experiences persistent or repeated ear problems, ventilating tubes may become necessary. Yet, this treatment program may strengthen his immune system and enable him to overcome his ear problems without surgery or the repeated use of antibiotics.

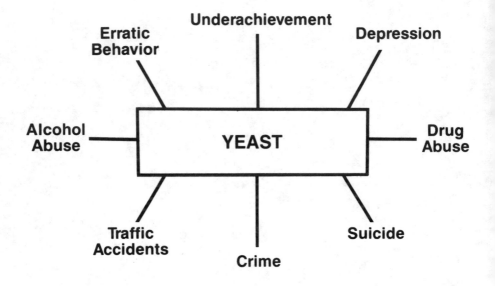

32
Physical And Mental Problems Of Teenagers

According to an article on May 26, 1983 by Mary Reed, Features Editor of my hometown paper, "The Jackson Sun,"

"A once carefree teenager, Chris Avrett, would spend some days sitting in one spot, depressed and oblivious to the world. At times he would be so disoriented he couldn't tie his shoe or get food to his mouth. After trips to physicians in Memphis, Jackson and Nashville, several hospital stays and $30,000 in medical bills, his parents still didn't have the answer to the cause or treatment for his problems."

Chris was referred to me on January 26, 1983 by Dr. Cheryl Robley, a clinical psychologist, who felt his problems could be related to candida. Chris gave a history of asthma and other allergies during his early years of life. Tubes were put in his ears when he was in the second grade and again in the fourth. He also had taken many antibiotics (especially the "broad spectrum" drugs which wipe out good germs along with the bad).

Like most youngsters, Chris loved sweets. Beginning at age 13, he changed from a happy boy who made good grades into a youngster with problems involving especially his nervous system . . . headache, anxiety, nervous twitching, short attention span and depression.

Continuing with Mary Reed's report,

"Peggy Avrett, Chris' mother, says that within a week of starting the diet and nystatin her son was much better. You wouldn't believe he was the same child, like daylight to dark. On the anti-yeast treatment his mother 'watched him go from being a helpless baby to his old self again'."

How many teenagers like Chris are "out there?" Could there be a yeast-connection to under-achievement in school? Or mental and nervous system disorders ranging from, nervous tics to severe depression? And how about alcoholism and other substance abuse, traffic accidents, crime and suicide? Could these perplexing disorders with multi-factoral causes also have a yeast connection?

I don't know, but my experiences during the past couple of years make me answer "Yes."

Tom (not his real name), a 17-year-old youngster enjoyed many economic, educational and cultural advantages. His parents were "super." They cared a lot. Tom was handsome, talented and smart.

Yet, Tom was depressed . . . very depressed . . . even suicidal. After spending two months in a special hospital for disturbed adolescents, he was put on an anti-yeast treatment program. He improved rapidly.

When Tom came in to see me on May 23, 1983, he looked great . . . absolutely radiant. And he was making plans for summer school so as to complete his college entrance requirements.

Tom commented,

> "If I cheat on my diet or don't take my medicine, I can feel my symptoms returning."

Candida isn't the only strand in the web of causes of teenage problems. Yet, several factors come into play in teenagers which can trigger the development of candida-related illness, including teenage acne, hormonal changes in teenagers (especially in girls) and ingestion or large amounts of sugar and yeast-containing foods.

Teenage Acne: Due to hormonal and other changes as the youngster matures, the oil glands of his face, chest and back become more active. And according to one report, 90% of all teenagers will show evidences of acne. Although most teenage acne will respond to soap and water and simple dietary changes, the "routine" treatment of more extensive teenage acne during the past two or three decades has included the use of antibiotics, especially tetracycline group of drugs, including Sumycin,® Panmycin,® Vibramycin® and Minocin.®

Recently I've seen a number of patients with severe candida-related problems who gave a history of long-term tetracycline treatment for acne and I submitted a clinical report on one such patient recently.[39]

I now feel that routine use of tetracycline in managing teenage acne

214

should be discontinued. And if, for any reason, tetracycline is prescribed for acne (or for any other condition), the Squibb preparation Mysteclin F® should be used, since it contains the anticandida drug, amphotericin B in combination with tetracycline.

Admittedly, acne troubles many teenagers and the condition is often difficult to manage. Yet, the risks of long-term tetracycline treatment are greater than the possible benefits. Moreover, if a teenager will eat a good diet and seek out the factors which promote good health, and avoid those factors which interfere with it, he'll usually be able to control and overcome his acne without resorting to potentially dangerous drugs.

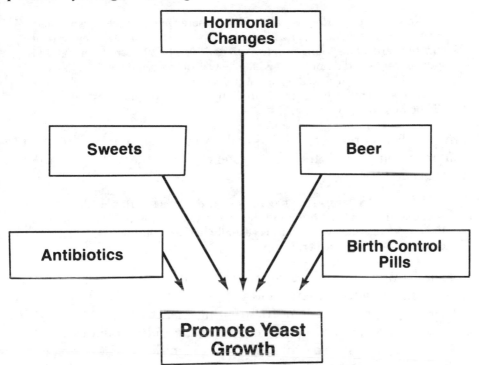

Hormonal Changes and "The Pill": When your child enters his teen years, all sorts of interrelated hormonal changes occur. His pituitary gland, like Rip Van Winkle, "wakes up." And it sends messages to other endocrine glands, including the thyroid, the adrenals and the sex glands (testicles or ovaries). These various glands also interact with each other.

These hormonal changes help turn your child into an adult. Yet, sometimes, the process isn't easy. Hormonal imbalances especially cause problems in the maturing female; and many girls are troubled by premenstrual tension, cramps, irregular periods, abdominal pain, headache, fatigue and other problems related to the menstrual cycle.

In some girls, these problems are severe enough to warrant consultation with a gynecologist. And many of these youngsters are put on birth control pills because of severe cramps or excessive bleeding.

As a result of the much talked about "sexual revolution", over half of American teenagers begin intercourse during their teen years. And several studies show that sexual activity begins in some ¼ to ⅓ of teenagers by the age of 15 or 16.

In discussing teen sex, Ann Landers[40] commented,

> "Recently on the Phil Donahue Show, there were two teenage mothers, one who had become pregnant at 13 and the other at 14 . . . They were attractive, articulate young people of 15 and 19. The 19 year old (her child is now 4) said she did not know what she was doing could result in having a baby. No one had talked to her about sex . . .
> "There were more than 1 million teenage pregnancies last year. Something is not working."

And in her continuing discussion Ann urged parents to "get a dialogue going" with their youngsters, giving them the information they need.

> "Very few teenagers stop having sex once they've started. Unless yours is one in five hundred thousand, he or she will continue. Once you have the knowledge that your child is sexually active, you must do what you can to protect him or her."

Helping and guiding teenagers (especially those who are sexually active) isn't easy for parents, and you or your physician may feel "the pill" is appropriate therapy for treating menstrual problems or for pregnancy prevention. However, since the pill stimulates candida, it's a two-edged sword which involves significant risks. So, in my opinion, alternate methods of pregnancy prevention should be sought.

Teenage Diet: As your youngsters grow up, you'll be astounded at how much they can eat . . . boys especially. They'll consume tremendous numbers of calories because they're growing so rapidly. I've seen teenage boys grow 6 inches and gain 30 pounds in a year. Many teenagers will eat anything that doesn't bite them first! Foods and beverages they like include pizza, candies, cakes, soft drinks and beer. All of these items are loaded with yeast and sugar.

Although many youngsters who consume these foods and beverages do not develop candida-related illness, such diets, especially when combined with hormonal changes, antibiotics, birth control pills and other antinutrient factors, lead to the development of candida-related health problems.

Although you may find it impossible to control your youngster's diet when he's away from home, offer him good foods when he is at home. What's more, good foods will contribute to the health of your entire family.

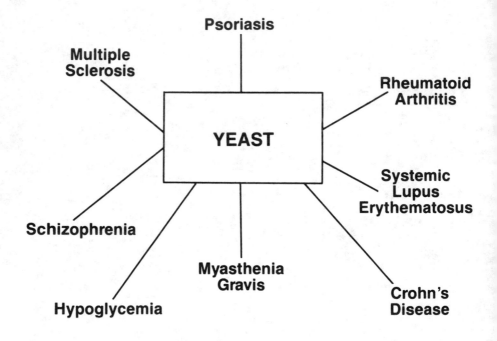

33

Does Candida Cause Multiple Sclerosis, Psoriasis, Arthritis Or Schizophrenia?

No—Candida isn't THE cause of these and other often devastating disorders including Crohn's disease (inflammation of the intestine), myasthenia gravis, systemic lupus erythematosus and some forms of hypoglycemia — but . . . there's growing evidence based on exciting clinical experiences of many physicians that there is a yeast connection.

And by treating the candida strand in the "Spider web" many individuals with these other disorders will start on the road to recovery.

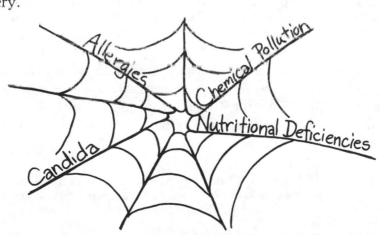

Bob, a 42-year-old soft drink executive, began to have twinges of pain in his left hand in March, 1982. It was worse if he struck his

219

hand against an object during his daily routines. Gradually, the pain, with associated numbness, involved his entire left arm. He then developed numbness and tingling in his left leg. Soon his left arm and leg became weak and he needed a cane for support.

Bob commented,

> "I have trouble knowing where my left arm and my leg are. And, at times, I've noticed tingling in my right buttock and thigh."

During the next few weeks his symptoms progressed and he was examined by a number of specialists in our town. In May, he was referred to a world famous clinic in the upper midwest for further observation and study. Here are excerpts from the medical report of the consultant who examined Bob:

> "Neurological exam revealed an ataxic, broad based, jerky gait. His deep tendon reflexes were brisk in both legs, more so on the left than the right . . . His reflexes in the left upper arm . . . were reduced . . . His muscle testing revealed mild left facial weakness and moderate weakness of the left upper extremities and mild weakness of the left lower extremity and right upper extremity. Muscle tone was increased in the left arm and both legs in a spastic fashion. There was some impairment of vibratory and joint sense in both the upper and lower extremities.
>
> *"It is our feeling that he has some type of demyelinating CNS disease. Whether this represents an acute episode of acute disseminating encephalomyelitis or a disease which will have recurrent episodes and be progressive cannot be determined at this time.* We told him that only future observation would confirm the diagnosis and that, in the case of acute flareups in the future, a short course of corticosteroids might be indicated. A long discussion was held with him and his wife and they seemed to understand fairly clearly the problem."

Bob came to see me in June, 1982. I prescribed an anti-candida program, including nystatin, a yeast-free, sugar-free, low carbohydrate diet, plus a variety of nutritional supplements (including essential fatty acids). He improved promptly and within six weeks he reported,

> "I can now play golf. All my symptoms are gone except for a little numbness and weakness in my left hand. I'm fine unless I cheat on my diet. *Even one bite of sugar-containing food will immediately trigger my symptoms.*"

In talking to Bob and his wife, they commented,

> "The doctors told us that Bob did indeed have multiple sclerosis and that the course was uncertain."

Bob comes in to see me at regular intervals and continues on his diet, nystatin, linseed oil and other nutritional supplements. In June, 1983 he commented, "I'm doing great."

Has Bob's severe neurological disease improved through coincidence, or has anticandida treatment helped?

Mutiple sclerosis is a disease that waxes and wanes, regardless of the sort of treatment used. Nevertheless, I feel the anticandida treatment has definitely helped Bob. Although I can't prove it, neither Bob nor his wife want to take a chance on discontinuing the anticandida program.

A similar patient, Ted, first came to me on October 1, 1982. Ted, a truck driver, had enjoyed general good health during his childhood, although he said,

> "I had a number of ear and throat infections and took a lot of antibiotics."

Then five years ago, he was involved in a serious accident and suffered extensive injuries. Treatment included insertion of an acrylic plate in his skull, plus lots of antibiotics.

Ted began to notice numbness, tingling and weakness in both of his feet and legs in December, 1981. He also experienced back pain and a loss of coordination. He was checked by a neurologist in March, 1982. The diagnosis: *multiple sclerosis.* Ted was checked at the same famous midwestern clinic in April, 1982. Here are excerpts from the report of his neurological examination:

> "His gait was slightly wide-based with circumduction of the right lower limb; there was mild tandem ataxia; there was mild static tremor in the hands bilaterally; coordination was slightly impaired in the left upper limb and alternate motion rate was minimally impaired in the left foot.
> "Mr. F. has demyelinating disease or multiple sclerosis. In view of the diagnosis, I suggest he strongly consider other types of work . . . I do not feel he should try to continue as a truck driver in view of the nature of his disease and the uncertain prognosis."

I prescribed a comprehensive program of management for Ted, including nystatin, a yeast free diet containing, initially, 100 grams of carbohydrates, essential fatty acid and vitamin/mineral supplements.

When I checked Ted one month later, he said,

>"I'm significantly better. The numbness, tingling and weakness are less intense. My incoordination is gone; my bladder problem and constipation are gone, my lower back pain is less intense."

At subsequent follow-up visits in December, 1982, February, 1983 and April, 1983, Ted has continued to do well. In December he commented,

>"I did show a little soreness after shoveling gravel. And I'm driving my truck about 10 thousand miles each month and have no symptoms of any sort unless I cheat on my diet and eat sweets or foods containing yeast."

Now I'd like to tell you about Dorothy, a 48 year old office worker I've known for 20 years. Here are excerpts from a letter she sent to me:

>"In 1969 I began taking sulfa drugs and I took them continuously for the next seven years to keep from developing infection related to kidney stones.
>"Beginning in 1975 I noticed that I was losing strength. My head hurt most of the time and I developed problems with my vision that would come and go. In 1977 I began to have joint pains. Yet, these too, would come and go. I was able to keep on working but I seemed to get weaker each year. In 1980 an eye doctor said I had scars in both eyes and in 1981 my left eye 'went out'. The doctor said it was optic neuritis."

In the 18 months before I saw Dorothy, she developed many strange sensations, including joint pains, numbness, tingling and "electricity" feeling in her legs, jerky handwriting, mental confusion, mood changes, headaches, bladder problems and eye symptoms. In addition, Dorothy commented,

>"At times I've felt I'd scream if I couldn't 'get out of my legs.' I felt like a person with boots on who needed to take them off. I also felt drugged and weak."

Dorothy was seen by several physicians, including an ophthalmologist and a neurologist. The neurologist told Dorothy,

>"It's possible you may be developing multiple sclerosis, although my findings on examination do not warrant my making such a diagnosis at this time."

Dorothy first came to me as a patient on June 14, 1982. In reviewing her history, the long-time consumption of sulfa drugs prior to the onset of her symptoms served as a "red flag". This history made me feel her health problems could be yeast-connected. So I prescribed a comprehensive program of management including nystatin, a yeast free, sugar free diet and nutritional supplements, including essential fatty acids. I saw her at monthly intervals and she showed consistent improvement.

On January 26, 1983, 7 months after beginning treatment, Dorothy commented,

> "Most of my major symptoms have disappeared, including mental confusion, headaches, numbness and weakness. I'm also pleased that most of the 'electricity feeling' in my arms and legs has disappeared. I still tire easily but this, too, is getting better."

Patients like Dorothy really excite me and make me say to myself,

> "Wouldn't it be great if patients with early MS-like symptoms could be turned around and made well before an actual 'disease' developed?"

Now I'd like to tell you about Phyllis, a slender 24-year-old office worker with a different sort of health problem. I first saw Phyllis on May 3, 1982. Her main complaints included "joint and muscle aches and pains, fatigue and depression." In a letter she commented:

> "For the last 4 years I've had aches and pains in every part of my body. Yet they weren't too severe until 5 months ago. Since then, they've been almost constant. The pains seem to travel from one part of my body to another. I also don't feel as active as I used to. I can't even scream . . . it seems as though I don't have enough breath."

When I reviewed Phyllis' history I found she was bothered by many other symptoms, including fatigue, depression, "peculiar feelings" in her ears, constant runny nose, sinus trouble, canker sores, dizziness, chest pains, nausea, frequent urination, irritability, numbness and tingling.

As a teenager, Phyllis took repeated antibiotics for "bladder infections." She also took birth control pills intermittently, beginning seven years ago, and had experienced vaginal yeast infections many times. Her diet included lots of junk foods including soft drinks. She also noted that exposure to perfumes and tobacco bothered her.

Three months before I first saw Phyllis, she had been comprehensively studied by a specialist in rheumatology. This physician examined her again in March, April and May, 1982, and here are excerpts from his medical report:

> "Phyllis continues to have polyarthritis, and in one instance had an episode of tenosynovitis of one wrist. She has a strongly positive FANA. Her anti-DNA antibodies were elevated at 42% and her serum complement is abnormal at 89 . . . *I therefore feel she probably has a definite rheumatoid arthritis without multi-system involvement.* Because of the increase in her symptoms, I've started her on Plaquenil®, 200 mgs. twice daily, and a trial of Feldene® at 20 mgs. each day."

On May 3, 1982, I put Phyllis on nystatin, ¼ teaspoon four times a day, and a yeast free diet with some carbohydrate restriction. A week later her anti-arthritic drugs were discontinued because of a severe skin rash involving especially her hands.

Within a few weeks, Phyllis began to improve and when I saw her again in October, 1982 she said,

> "I'm much better. However, certain foods disagree with me and make my joint pains worse, including yeasts, wheat, sugar, milk, potatoes and beef."

I instructed Phyllis to avoid the foods that caused trouble, to rotate her diet and to continue her nystatin, vitamins and minerals. I also prescribed calcium and magnesium complex.

When Phyllis returned on April 19, 1983 for a review visit, she said,

> "I've improved 100% since starting on my anti-yeast program. What's more, I was checked by my internist and all my blood tests are now normal. I still stay away from perfumes and smokes, and I have to be careful about my diet. I find if I take ½ teaspoon of nystatin at each dose, I feel better."

Credit for first recognizing the relationship of Candida albicans to patients with severe mental and neurological manifestations goes to Dr. C. Orian Truss. And in his first paper[51a] presented in the spring of 1977, Dr. Truss told of six patients with severe health problems who improved on anti-yeast therapy, including small doses of candida extract and nystatin.

One of his patients was a 36 year old woman who had been treated for schizophrenia for six years.

"After many courses of drug and electroshock therapy, her condition had deteriorated to the point that permanent commitment to the state mental hospital had been recommended by her psychiatrist . . . This woman was treated for one year with nothing other than the Candida albicans extract. Followup ten years later found her well."

(A second patient)

. . . "A young white woman was relatively free of health problems until 24 years of age. Then after taking tetracycline, She promptly developed yeast vaginitis which recurred intermittently during the next three years."

This patient also

". . . began to have episodes of marked abdominal distention, associated with anxiety and depression."

Premenstrual tension also became a severe problem.

Dr. Truss treated her with oral nystatin and her symptoms, including anxiety and depression, vanished.

Another patient, a 30 year old woman, developed a visual field defect in November, 1972. A year later, she developed numbness and tingling of both lower extremities.

"The diagnosis of multiple sclerosis was made and discussed with the patient by her neurologist . . ."

In discussing this patient, Dr. Truss commented,

"Again, the total picture is one of lifelong allergy, chronic intestinal and vaginal symptoms, and poor hormone function. Many courses of antibiotic were administered from childhood on The initial neurological symptom occurred during massive antibiotic therapy over a four-month period for the severe lung infection." . . . "After two years of nystatin therapy neurological examination was 'entirely normal'."

In his third paper, "The Role of Candida Albicans in Human Illness,"[51c] presented in September, 1981, Dr. Truss briefly described the successful treatment of several patients with severe and often devastating health problems. One of these was the 30-year-old woman he had reported in his first paper.

"She is entirely well now, seven years after nystatin was begun. She went through pregnancy with no trouble and delivered a normal baby."

He also told of several other patients with multiple sclerosis who improved on anti-candida therapy. One of these, like my patient, Bob, was a 31-year-old woman who started . . . "improving immediately" on nystatin and who would remain asymptomatic unless she went "on a carbohydrate binge."

Dr. Truss also told of one case of Crohn's disease which cleared, and he commented,

> "I know of two additional different auto-immune diseases, systemic lupus erythematosus and thrombocytopenic purpura, that have responded."

At the Informal Conference on Candida Albicans in July, 1982, the relationship of multiple sclerosis and other severe auto-immune diseases was discussed by the participants in attendance. Many physicians reported successful experiences in treating patients with these disorders with an anti-candida program. Yet, a number of participants pointed out that other factors played a role in causing such illnesses. They also emphasized that individuals with severe auto-immune diseases, including those with multiple sclerosis who had been confined to wheel chairs for years, could anticipate little benefit from anti-candida therapy.

To obtain current information about the experiences of other physicians I sent out a questionnaire in March, 1983. One question asked, "How many patients with multiple sclerosis, lupus, arthritis, Crohn's disease or other auto-immune disease have you successfully treated using an anti-candida program?

One physician listed two patients with Crohn's disease and one with multiple sclerosis. Another physician listed one patient with Crohn's disease "who did well." One physician commented,

> "These diseases are multi-factoral. The candida approach only seems to play a part."

Another physician commented,

> "I can't answer this question, as I never treat these patients with just yeast eradication. However, I often start treatment with yeast eradication and many patients show significant improvement. Yet, I've rarely seen a patient who could correct the total disease process of a yeast eradication program alone."

Other physicians have found that patients with multiple sclerosis and other severe auto-immune diseases can be helped by an anti-candida program. Dr. E. W. Rosenberg, Professor and Chairman, Division of Dermatology, University of Tennessee Center for the Health Sciences in Memphis, recently described the successful treatment of psoriasis by a program designed to get rid of gut yeast. Here are excerpts from Dr. Rosenberg's letter in a recent issue of "The New England Journal of Medicine:[41]

> ". . . We have become aware . . . of improvement of both psoriasis and inflammatory bowel disease in patients treated with oral nystatin, an agent that was expected to work only on yeasts in the gut lumen. We have now confirmed that observation in several of our patients with psoriasis. We suspect, therefore, that gut yeast may have a role in some instances of psoriasis."

Does candida cause multiple sclerosis, psoriasis, arthritis, schizophrenia and other devastating auto-immune diseases?

No, candida isn't *the* cause.

Yet, there's growing evidence, based on the clinical experiences of many physicians, that the yeast organism, *Candida albicans*, is an important strand in the "web" of causes of these and other diseases.

34

Can Candida Albicans Make A "Tee-totaler" Drunk?

According to a syndicated article† by Don G. Campbell from the Los Angeles Times News Service, January, 1983, Candida albicans played a role in making "poor old Charlie Swaart" drunk, even though no alcohol had touched his lips. According to the article, Charlie Swaart was picked up for drunk driving following a dinner-theater party given by a prominent Arizona politician. Yet, he hadn't been drinking. "He had a 'still' in his intestines that was capable of converting carbohydrates directly into alcohol."

In thousands of "binges" spanning 30 years, Charlie Swaart would become "a sloppy, overbearing and hostile . . . sometimes even violent . . . drunk," even though he hadn't consumed any alcohol.

"Swaart's bouts were straining his private and professional life." Then, in the mid-1960's, a clue emerged that "nature was playing a cruel trick on Charlie." On a rigid, high protein, low carbohydrate diet prescribed to curb weight, Charlie's episodes of drunkenness decreased. Then a friend gave him an article in an old (July 20, 1959) issue of *Time* magazine. This reprint told of a 46-year-old Japanese, Kozo Ohishi, and his 25-year binge that brought him social and professional disgrace and a besmirched army record.

According to the *Time* article, Ohishi was studied at Hokkaido University Hospital in Japan where samples were taken of his digestive juices. In them, microbiologists found a flourishing growth of a yeast-like fungus, *Candida albicans.* When treated with a Japanese anti-candida drug, trichomycin, Ohishi stayed sober.

---

† "The Ordeal of 'Poor Old Charlie,' Drinkless Drunk" by Don G. Campbell. Copyright, 1983, Los Angeles Times. Used by permission.

Swaart's Phoenix physician ordered tests "and they showed massive colonies of the yeasts" in his intestines . . . "His subsequent research established that about 60% of the population has some yeast in the alimentary canal, and that this yeast is capable of producing some alcohol in the stomach, but never to the level of intoxication.

Swaart was then treated with mycostatin (nystatin) and improved. However, "In 1970, the mycostatin began losing its punch, and the symptoms returned — with a vengeance."

Although 30 Japanese victims, ranging in age from 3 to 74, had been identified, Swaart was the first non-Japanese to be stricken with these peculiar candida-related health problems. So Dr. Kazuo Iwata, the professor of microbiology at the University of Tokyo School of Medicine, came by to visit Swaart at his Phoenix home. Cultures and microscopic examinations of Swaart's intestinal contents showed he had a "raging case" of *meitei-sho*†.

But Swaart ran into a problem. "The drugs recommended by Iwata and found effective in Tokyo had not been approved by the Food and Drug Administration and were not available in the United States."

Swaart's problems continued until he flew to Tokyo where studies were done which showed that a new antifungal drug developed by Hoffman-La Roche in Switzerland was effective in helping him overcome his problem.

Since the drug wasn't available in the United States, he brought a year's supply home with him. This drug discouraged the growth of candida in Charlie's intestines. After taking the drug for some months, he was able to discontinue it in September, 1975.††

---

† *Meitei-sho* is the name given by the Japanese to the syndrome of intoxication due to candida in the gut. *Meitei* means *drunk*; *sho* means *disease*. Hence, in Japanese: "drunk disease".

†† In a recent letter to me, Charlie Swaart pointed out that *Meitei-sho* can recur, especially if a person takes antibiotics. Charlie stated, "To save my life during a pneumonia episode, doctors gave me antibiotrics . . . I got up from my pneumonia sick bed to fall flat on my face with a *Meitei-sho* return . . . This syndrome can be controlled . . . prevented . . . and attacks avoided, but the problem of freedom from candida intoxication . . . once you've been a *Meitei-sho* victim, is eternal vigilance."

Swaart pointed out that *Meitei-sho* isn't rare and that he and his wife had received hundreds of telephone calls and letters from people all over the world describing similar *Meitei-sho* attacks. "In your book, you could be a great service by alerting the medical profession of the fact that my case is NOT a 'medical curiosity' but a candida syndrome that . . . is no longer confined to Japan."

35

Overcoming Yeast-Connected Illness Isn't Always Easy

Helping people overcome yeast-connected health problems has made my life interesting, challenging, rewarding and exciting. Some 90 percent of the hundreds of my patients with yeast connected illness have improved. Many a patient reports,

> "I'm well. No problems. And I can even cheat on my diet without triggering symptoms."

Although each patient differs from every other patient, most have been helped by the comprehensive program of management described in Sections A, B, C, and F of this book.

Because of the favorable response, I feel confident that if you're bothered by yeast connected health problems, *you, too, will improve and you can ultimately get well.* So I urge you to take the steps needed to accomplish such a goal.

But conquering yeast-connected health problems isn't always easy. And not all of my patients improved immediately . . . or even in a few months. Moreover, some who improved initially relapsed and an occasional patient became worse. Although diet, nystatin, nutritional supplements and avoiding environmental molds and chemicals help most of my patients, some have had to struggle with their problems for months or years after starting treatment. Since most of the people I've told you about in this book are "success stories," I feel I should present the "other side of the coin."

Forty-one year old Sandra first came to see me in April, 1980. Here are excerpts from her 4-page letter:

"I've been married for almost 22-years, and for 15-years I've been bothered by persistent vaginal yeast infection. For at least 10-years I've had to make myself get out of bed every morning. I couldn't hear alarm clocks, so my husband would literally have to drag me out of bed. I feel tired and dazed, like a rag doll or a wet wash rag . . . I think I could sleep 24-hours a day and still feel sleepy and tired.

Over the years I've been to all sorts of doctors because of my many complaints, including aching in my neck, joints and legs, bronchitis, nervousness, weakness, rectal itching, noises in my ears, constipation, bloating . . . I get so depressed I've thought about taking my own life.

I've been hospitalized several times, but the tests never seemed to show anything. Chemicals of all sorts bother me, including several brands of perfume and air freshener. Also, my symptoms get worse when I eat sweetened foods or drink milk."

Because of her "typical history", I put Sandra on "the program", including diet, nystatin, nutritional supplements, environmental control and immunotherapy. She has steadily improved, although there have been ups and downs. And after more than three years of treatment, she continues to experience problems.

At a visit in June, 1983, Sandra said,

"I'm still taking my nystatin and I occasionally take small doses of Nizoral® which always seems to help. Yet, when I cheat on my diet, my symptoms always flare. Although I feel a lot better than I felt three years ago, many symptoms continue to bother me. Rainy weather makes my joints and legs hurt and I'm still bothered by chemicals. Just going to the grocery store 'wipes me out' and I go into a drug-like sleep when I get home."

A second patient, 31-year old Karen, a registered nurse and mother of four, first came to see me on October 1, 1981. And because her history illustrates so many important points, I'm reproducing in full a letter she wrote me November 19, 1982, 13-months after she started on a comprehensive program of treatment:

"As I write about my problems with yeast-related illness, I've been properly diagnosed and on anti-candida treatment for over a year. All of my symptoms aren't gone, but I'm confident that continuing my prescribed treatment plan will some day get me well.

"As a child, I took many unneeded *antibiotics* for colds and well-meaning neighbors provided me with too much *candy*. Knowing what I know now, I feel both of these factors set the stage for my long battle with *vaginal problems.*

"Trouble with *menstrual cramps* began when I started my period at age 12. But after my first *yeast infection* at age 17, my cramps became severe

232

enough to spend a day in bed every month. And during the week before each period, I was irritable, bloated and generally miserable.

"I began on birth control pills a month before my marriage at age 19. I took them for three months, but felt so bad I had to discontinue them. I promptly became *pregnant* and was bothered by *cystitis* and *vaginal yeast infections* throughout my pregnancy.

"The next 2½ years brought two more pregnancies, one of which was spontaneously aborted. During this time I was treated with antibiotics for 10 episodes of *'cystitis.'* Recently, my doctor commented, 'Many of your symptoms were probably caused by candida irritation of your bladder outlet . . . the urethra.'

"I also experienced *joint pains and swelling,* involving especially my knees. And I was given *cortisone* and other steroids on several occasions. I began to notice, for the first time, that getting around odorous cleaning materials made me sick.

"Then early in my third pregnancy, I had my first *migraine headache* and I had no idea that it could be related to diet and my other problems.

"After the birth of my second child, I took *birth control pills* for seven months, but once again I had to stop them because I felt worse than I'd ever felt in my life. My *vaginitis* continued and my *cystitis* was so severe that my gynecologist sent me to a urologist.

"I was put on a *broad-spectrum antibiotic* for six weeks and told to take antibiotics 'for the rest of my life' . . . anytime I had urgency and frequency for several days in a row.

"At the age of 25, my *migraine headaches* became so severe that I consulted a neurosurgeon. Various drugs were prescribed to control the migraines. Yet these drugs caused so many side-effects and so much emotional upset that I soon stopped them.

"About that time, I saw another gynecologist to see if he could help me control my *vaginal infections.* Although he was kind during my first visit, he finally lost his patience and told me "not to bother him" with something as unimportant as vaginal infections! He told me I'd have to learn to live with them.

"My *fourth pregnancy* at age 26 put more pressures on what I now realize was my *weakened immune system.* I was given *progesterone* for an irritable uterus and while I was taking it my vaginal problems were aggravated. And as I've since learned, pregnancy also worsens vaginal yeast problems.

"I went into labor at around 32 weeks and was given intravenous alcohol and *steroids.* Soon afterward, I experienced severe burning in my throat, esophagus and stomach which lasted for 5 months and kept me depressed and very uncomfortable.

"I also experienced *visual disturbances,* along with *abdominal bloating* and *constipation.* My *fatigue* was full-blown by now, but I attributed it to having a new baby.

"I also noticed that turning on the *gas heat* that winter triggered my *migraine* headaches and I remember saying to myself, 'it seems crazy to think the gas heat is making me sick'. Little did I know.

"Something I haven't mentioned before is the increased *craving for sweets* which I developed over a period of many years. And during my fifth pregnancy, at age 27, I ate plenty of good foods but added a lot of junk food, too. My *visual disturbances, fatigue* and *vaginal problems* were all prominent during this pregnancy. However, after the baby was born, I began eating a high protein, low carbohydrate diet which temporarily relieved some of my symptoms.

"Then at the age of 28, all of my previous symptoms either returned or became more prominent and I experienced many new ones, including *headache* and *severe abdominal pain.* This pain was so bad that my husband took me to the doctor on two occasions because he thought I had appendicitis.

"In the meantime, my *ability to concentrate decreased,* my *memory became worse* and I got up every morning *tired.* My *vaginal symptoms* of pain, burning, itching and heavy discharge were full-blown. I was taking *antibiotics* all the time as well as using different vaginal creams and suppositories. Nothing helped me and I became increasingly miserable.

"My *depression* became a real problem and I cried so easily for seemingly no reason, and my premenstrual tension became worse. My husband was very supportive and that helped. He would assure me that I wasn't 'crazy.' (Now that I'm better, he commented recently, 'I really thought I was going to lose you.')

"My gynecologist was kind and tried everything he knew to do. I hate to admit it now, but some days the thought of death was pleasant. The only thing that helped me get through many days was memorizing the Psalms of the Bible. As I cried, I'd quote the scriptures and I'd get hope to go on.

"At the age of 29, I had a *hysterectomy.* Some of my backache and abdominal pain improved for a while, and the premenstrual symptoms were gone. However, other symptoms developed, including *numbness and tingling of my extremities,* daily *visual problems, excessive intestinal gas* and throat mucus, *joint pain* and *heart palpitations.*

"I kept a *headache* that never left. Sometimes it was mild, at other times it was severe. I felt so horrible I would pray, 'Lord, Jesus, how can I keep living this way?' My gynecologist continued to be supportive, but I never told him of my many symptoms for fear he'd send me to a psychiatrist.

"Then in October, 1981, through a sort of unique coincidence (it was definitely an answer to my prayers), I first learned about yeast-related illness. Soon afterward, I was put on a comprehensive treatment program to help me get rid of candida, improve my immune system and regain my health.

"Many different things have helped me, including nystatin, Nizoral® and the yeast free, low carbohydrate diet. Allergy vaccines for inhalants, foods and candida have also been essential parts of my treatment program. I've also been helped by nutritional supplements, including essential fatty acids, minerals and vitamins. A blood study sent to the Medical College of New Jersey (New Jersey Medical School, 88 Ross St., East Orange, New Jersey 07018) showed I was low in vitamin A, even though I'd been taking a multiple vitamin preparation containing supposedly adequate amounts of all the vitamins. Reducing my exposure to chemicals has also helped.

"Today, November 19, 1982, my vaginal symptoms are better but they are still present and bothersome. However, all the other problems are gone all or most of the time. I feel better than I have in many years and I'm grateful for the answer to my prayers."

Karen came in for a review visit on December 21, 1982. She commented,

"I'm slowly getting better, but I still have my 'ups and downs.' Nystatin douches help my vaginitis, but the symptoms never go away and I must take tremendous doses of nystatin to control them . . . the equivalent of 48 to 50 tablets a day. I wish I could take Nizoral® again, it really helped last year. My candida shots in the weak dilutions help most of the time and I take them two or three times a week."

I continued Karen on the same basic program with a few modifications and changes. Because her liver enzymes had returned to normal, I added a small dose of Nizoral® to her treatment program . . . ¼ tablet twice a week. Mold cultures of her home showed that the mold, *hormodendrum,* was the principle offender. Appropriate changes were then made in Karen's extracts.

Karen returned for another visit on February 9, 1983. She commented,

"I was involved in an automobile accident in January. I received many bruises and had to have a lot of x-rays. Although I experienced no serious injuries, I've been worse since the accident. I've had more vaginal burning and my fatigue level is high again. I was also bothered by a rash on two different days last week."

After reviewing Karen's treatment program, I suggested the following additional things which I hoped would help:

1. Laxative as needed to keep her colon cleaned out and hopefully get rid of some of the candida.
2. Enemas containing ½ to 1 teaspoon of nystatin to ½ pint of water. (A report from a Florida patient plus research studies from several sources indicate that candida colonization is greatest in the colon. Accordingly, reaching and killing these organisms from below would appear especially appropriate.)
3. Because I'd also learned that the Squibb preparation, amphotericin B (see pages 257-260) was available in France and Switzerland, I made arrangements to obtain some of this preparation to see if it would help. I also discontinued the Nizoral®.

On March 28, 1983, Karen again returned. Here are a few of her comments:

"That automobile accident really set me back. My vaginitis continues to bother me and my fatigue level remains high. My prescription for amphotericin B was filled by a French pharmacy and sent to me a couple of weeks ago. I started taking it, but so far it hasn't helped."

On May 16, 1983, Karen reported,

"I'm improving and I've finally gotten back to where I was before my accident in January. My fatigue and joint pains are better although on damp days when the mold count is high, I don't feel as good. I'm continuing the oral and vaginal amphotericin B. I dump the contents of 1 capsule in my mouth four times daily and insert the powder from 1 capsule into my vagina twice daily. This seems to work better than nystatin in doses of over a teaspoon of powder four times daily. (For a discussion of amphotericin B, see pages 257-260.)

"I'm also following all of the other parts of the comprehensive program of management you prescribed, including inhalant and food vaccines, linseed oil, primrose oil and other nutritional supplements. I also have restricted my diet to meats, eggs and vegetables for the past 10 days but can't tell that leaving off fruits and grains has made a significant difference.

"So to repeat, I'm really doing well with all symptoms except the vulvovaginitis which continues to cause varying degrees of discomfort and frustration."

On January 3, 1984, Karen commented,

"Everything is better. I'm even free of vaginal pain and discomfort most of the time. I feel great, lots lof energy and none of the other symptoms I used to have unless I cheat on my diet. And I did cheat during the holidays and had brownies. Within twelve hours, I developed bladder urgency, frequency and pain, even though I found I don't have an infection. Also, I still can't tolerate perfumes, chemicals or mold exposure.

My next two patients came to see me early in 1983. The first of these, 31-year old Sue, first consulted me on February 8, 1983. Here are excerpts from the long letter she wrote:

"My health problems began many years ago. During my high school years I was bothered by headaches and sore throats; while in college, I developed bladder infections which have recurred many times. Nevertheless, I felt good most of the time.

"Immediately after graduation from college in May, 1974, I began working with a fascinating company and I continue to work for them. In July, 1974 I was married and from that time on I've been going down hill. First it was just one small illness after another and in between I felt OK. However, I began to feel tired most of the time. I was bothered by abdominal symptoms which were diagnosed as "spastic colon." During the year I was constantly plagued by one thing after another. Incidentally, I had begun taking birth control pills.

"By the spring of 1975, I was taken off the pill and I seemed to get better for a time, but then my headaches and sinus troubles returned. Allergy testing showed sensitivity to molds and weeds. I took injections for several years but they didn't really help. Meanwhile, my general health deteriorated, with headaches, sore throats and general aches and pains. All of my friends would joke and call me 'sickly Sue'. I never felt good.

"In 1979, during my pregnancy, my headaches increased in frequency and severity. I also experienced my first vaginal yeast infection and kept it for months. Worst of all, I began having bouts of fast heart beat (the doctors called it 'paroxysmal tachycardia'). For a time after my baby was born, I felt better for a couple of months but then my fatigue returned. Most of the time I ached all over and kept a sore throat. During the years, 1980-81, I was taking antibiotics almost constantly, including Terramycin®, Vibramycin®, Panmycin®, ampicillin, Keflex® and Septra®. Finally, in March, 1982 my tonsils were removed. Infections continued.

"During the past couple of years, I've been given all sorts of tests, including cardiograms, x-rays and a glucose tolerance test. The latter test resulted in a diagnosis of 'hypoglycemia'.

"Six weeks ago, my headaches took on a new dimension. The only thing I had done differently was to take a lot of a 'health-energy protein drink' which I later found contained yeast. I'm at a loss as to what's wrong with me, and I continue to have headaches, tachycardia and fatigue. I'm susceptible to every germ that comes along. I go to bed tired and wake up tired. I can sleep half the day away when the opportunity arises. Please help me get well.'"

Because of her typical history, I put Sue on the anticandida program, including diet, nystatin and nutritional supplements.
On March 15th, Sue said

"I'm a little better, although my headaches still come and go."

In May she reported,

"I'm still experiencing many problems and although I'm improving, all of my symptoms bother me."

Sue returned for a comprehensive checkup on July 5, 1983. And in a treatment diary she commented,

"I work every day and I'm a productive person. Yet, I'm struggling. I worry because I weigh 5 pounds less than when I started. Headaches are still my major symptoms and weakness and bouts of tachycardia continue, even though I've been taking ½ teaspoon of nystatin four times a day and eating mainly meats and vegetables."

Because of Sue's persistent problems, in spite of 5 months on 'the program,' I prescribed Nizoral®. In addition, because her morning temperature readings were only 96.5° to 97° (in spite of normal thyroid tests), I also prescribed a half grain of thyroid once daily. (See also pages 251-252.) Then because Sue said,

> "Several foods, including eggs and beef bother me; yet I feel I need to eat these foods to keep from wasting away,"

I scheduled Sue for food testing and possible immunotherapy with food extracts. (See also pages 252-254.)

Another recent patient, Matilda, a 50-year old teacher was first seen on February 11, 1983. Here are excerpts from her 8-page letter:

> "Since September, 1980, I've been trapped in a cycle of chronic pain and intermittent depression. I've taken all sorts of medicines, including antibiotics, tranquillizers, pain pills and decongestants. My symptoms, including pain in my head and legs, anger and mood swings became so frightening, I saw a psychotherapist. I went to other physicians including a gynecologist who said my symptoms were "menopausal." In addition, I've been troubled by recurrent vaginal yeast infections, abdominal pain and extreme fatigue, and exposure to chemicals, especially fabric shop odors, causes severe symptoms."

Because of her typical history, I put Matilda on a comprehensive treatment program including nystatin, diet and nutritional supplements. At a follow-up visit two weeks later, Matilda reported,

> "I've had my ups and downs. One exciting thing . . . my ears stopped ringing. However, I continue to be bothered by strange "thinking disturbances" and hallucinations at night."

Nystatin and diet were continued. At a visit in March, Matilda said,

> "Although my upper respiratory symptoms are better, my cerebral symptoms are bad and my chemical sensitivity is severe. I itch all over my body. I'm wondering if my dentures and fixed bridges could contribute to my problem, since my gums have been bleeding."

At a followup visit on April 22, Matilda said,

"I've increased my nystatin to ½ teaspoon four times a day; yet this causes a lot of 'die-off' symptoms."

At a visit on May 15, she reported,

"My vaginitis continues to cause severe discomfort even though I'm staying on my diet, taking nystatin and using vaginal suppositories. Four or five days ago I was so confused I was running around town like a frightened rabbit. Perhaps it was related to my premenstrual hormones. I got better when I started my period."

Because of Matilda's continuing severe symptoms, including 'die-off' symptoms from nystatin, on May 15th I prescribed Nizoral®. At a visit on May 23, Matilda said,

"I couldn't tolerate the Nizoral®, it caused severe burning in my stomach. Damp days make me feel terrible. My house also makes me sick, especially since my husband continues to smoke. I really need to be in a hospital. *I feel terribly discouraged.*"

I encouraged Matilda to "Stay the course" and to continue with her diet, nystatin, environmental control and nutritional supplements. I hope she'll soon improve. Yet, like several of my other patients with complex problems who live in homes or areas contaminated by high levels of chemicals or molds, she may have to move or make drastic changes in her home in order to improve significantly.

It should now be obvious that health problems in people with yeast connected illness are related to a *weakened immune system.* Or, putting it in simple terms, *"lowered resistance."*

In most patients with these disorders, illness develops over a period of many months and years. Moreover, the causative factors tend to be multiple and complex.

Strengthening the immune system and regaining health may occasionally be quick and easy. *More often, it takes time, patience, persistence and careful management of the multiple factors contributing to the illness.*

Section
E

Other
helpful
information

36

Miscellaneous Measures That May Help You

If you're bothered by yeast-connected illness and are taking nystatin and following the *Candida Control Diet* and your symptoms continue to bother you, what else can you do? Here are comments and suggestions I've obtained from various sources, including my patients and other physicians:

1. *Low Carbohydrate Diet:* Carbohydrates of any type, even the good ones, may promote candida growth in your digestive tract. If you do not improve on the Candida Control Diet, try the Low Carbohydrate Diet for 4 weeks or longer (see pages 75-93. Or try the Fruit-free, Grain-free, Milk-free, Nut-free diet (see page 119)

2. *Hidden Food Allergies:* Adverse or allergic reactions to any food, including such protein foods as milk, egg, beef or soy, may be contributing to your health problems. To identify such food troublemakers, try the "cave man" diet for a week and see if your symptoms get better. Then add back the eliminated foods, one at a time, and see if your symptoms worsen. (You'll find complete instructions for carrying out this diet in my book, *Tracking Down Hidden Food Allergy*,[13] pages 25-38 and 49-53.).

3. *Rotated Diets:* If you're eating the same food every day, you may develop an intolerance or allergy to that food. To keep this from happening, rotate your diet (see pages 129-130).

4. *Multivitamin and Mineral Supplements:* Take a yeast free, sugar free, color free vitamin/mineral preparation. Preparations I use contain extra amounts of the B vitamins, 300 to 1500 mgs. of vitamin C, 15 mgs. of zinc and other supplemen-

243

tal nutrients. (These preparations are available from many different companies.) *READ LABELS CAREFULLY* to make sure the preparation contains no yeast.

5. *Vitamin C:*

a. Time release vitamin C capsules, 500 mgs. twice daily.

b. Vitamin C powder. In general, there are two main forms . . . ascorbic acid and a buffered form including calcium ascorbate. A teaspoon of these powders contains 3500 to 4000 milligrams of vitamin C. I've found that vitamin C in large doses (2000 to 20,000 mgs. or more daily) helps many of my pa-tients with immune system problems. Included among these patients are those with yeast-connected illness. The total dose can be monitored by using the "bowel tolerance" test of Cathcart[54] and Pauling[21].

In discussing the usage of large doses of vitamin C. Dr. Pauling commented, saying in effect,

> "Persons with viral infections or under other types of stress can take gradually increasing doses of vitamin C to strengthen the immune system. If and when the vitamin C causes diarrhea or digestive upset, the dose can be decreased."

Norman Cousins, in his book, *Anatomy of an Illness,*[31] describes his own personal experiences with large doses of vitamin C. Mr. Cousins took 25,000 mgs. of vitamin C each day for a number of days and his physicians felt this therapy played a significant role in his recovery from a severe illness. One of my colleagues, Susan Karlgaard, commented,

> "I take 5,000 to 20,000 mgs. of vitamin C every day. I find it especially helps when I've been exposed to chemicals or when I've eaten the wrong food.".

A 13-year-old patient (I'll call him Harvey) with severe asthma came in with an attack of wheezing in March, 1983. This youngster had been hospitalized many times and had received all types of therapy from pediatricians, allergists, and pulmonary specialists. Harvey's skin tests showed sharp reactions to many environmental inhalants, including especially molds. He was also sensitive to a number of foods and received many antibiotics and courses of steroids. He was taking regular, around-the-clock bronchodilators, immunotherapy, cromolyn solution inhalations, nystatin and a yeast free diet, with intermittent injections of Adrenalin® and Susphrine®.

In spite of these measures, he was experiencing increasing difficulty during the two days prior to his visit to me. He and his mother were reluctant to go back on prednisone or enter the hospital for more intensive therapy.

I increased Harvey's nystatin from 1/8 teaspoon four times daily to ½ teaspoon (2-million units) each dose, and, out of desperation and more or less as a "shot in the dark," I decided to try him on large doses of vitamin C. I instructed his mother to get vitamin C powder containing 1 part ascorbic acid and 1 part calcium ascorbate . . . 4,000 mgs. per teaspoon . . . and to give Harvey 1 teaspoon in a glass of water every 1 to 2 hours if tolerated.

Harvey took 35,000 mgs. of vitamin C by mouth for each of the next three days. His wheezing began to improve in 12 hours and cleared by the end of 48 hours and no further injections of Adrenalin® were required. By the end of the third day, Harvey's stools became loose and his dose of vitamin C was decreased to 10,000 to 15,000 mgs. per day. When rechecked two weeks later, he was being continued on this same dose and his mother commented,

"The vitamin C really made a difference."

In a follow-up conversation with Harvey's mother on May 18, 1983, she commented,

"Even though we're right in the middle of the grass pollen season, Harvey is doing great . . . at least great for him. He's outdoors every day running and playing. He is even planning to run in a mile race. He's still taking 12,000 mgs. of vitamin C each day plus his nystatin, cromolyn and Vaponefrin® inhalations and immunotherapy.

On July 15, 1983, I received the following report:

"Harvey continues to do exceedingly well and is going to camp for the first time in his life. The nystatin and vitamin C truly make a difference. Other therapies, including his cromolyn and Vaponefrin®, had never controlled his wheezing until he began on big doses of nystatin and vitamin C. Also, if he forgets to take either his nystatin or vitamin C, he notices chest tightness.

"Something else of interest is my other 5 children came down with a bad virus . . . high fever and vomiting. One had to be hospitalized. Yet, Harvey didn't get sick. I think the nystatin and vitamin C may have strengthened his immune system."

6. *Calcium and magnesium supplements:* Unless you take dairy products, salad greens, clams or oysters on a regular basis, chances are you aren't getting enough calcium. I recommend supplemental calcium in a dose of 1000 to 1500 milligrams a day, along with 400 to 600 milligrams of magnesium.

Over the years, I've recommended a number of different types of calcium and magnesium preparations, including bone meal and dolomite. However, several recent studies suggest that some of these preparations may contain worrisome quantities of lead. Yet, *Prevention* magazine reported that the lead content of bone meal and dolomite preparations they examined contained no more lead than ordinary fruits and vegetables. Nevertheless, I prefer calcium and magnesium preparations derived from other sources. (See, also, page 138.)

7. *Essential fatty acids:* Unprocessed oils, including especially evening primrose oil and linseed oil, contain vital nutrients, including GLA (gamma-linolenic acid) and CLA (cis-linoleic acid). Your body needs these substances to make a family of hormone-like compounds called *prostaglandins.* These substances play a vital role in controlling normal functions of every organ of the body.

You can obtain evening primrose oil in capsule form from many pharmacies and most health food stores. The recommended dose is 1 or 2 capsules two to three times a day. Linseed oil can also be obtained from most health food stores and I recommend 1 to 2 tablespoons a day.† It can be combined with freshly squeezed lemon juice and used for salad dressing.

You can learn more about essential fatty acids from the pamphlet, "Evening Primrose Oil," by Richard A. Passwater, Ph.D., published by Keats Publishing Co., Inc., 35 Grove St. (Box 876), New Canaan, Connecticut 06840, and from a fascinating article by David Horrobin, Ph.D. in the June, 1981 *Executive Health* (Pickfair Bldg., Rancho Santa Fe, California 92067).

8. *Iron Supplements:* Such supplements may help you even if you aren't anemic. (See also page 138.) However, iron sup-

---

†According to Dr. Donald Rudin, some individuals are sensitive to tablespoon-size amounts of linseed oil. Yet they respond favorably to ½-1 teaspoon of the oil twice daily.

plements should not be continued indefinitely and should be prescribed by your physician.

9. *Intravaginal nystatin:* Candida makes its home on all of the mucous membranes of the body, including the vagina. Even if you aren't bothered by vaginal symptoms, use intravaginal nystatin once or twice daily or a suppository containing anticandida medication. Here's a convenient and economical way to accomplish this: After your bath, moisten your finger and coat it with 1/8 teaspoon of nystatin, then insert it high into your vagina. Other intravaginal, anti-candida medications are also available, including Gyne-Lotrimin®, Monistat-7® suppositories or cream and Mycelex G® cream.

10. *Sniffing or inhaling nystatin:* Many patients can clear nasal congestion, postnasal drip and mental and nervous symptoms by inhaling nystatin. Here's how you do it: Shake your bottle of nystatin powder vigorously. Remove the cap and hold the bottle just under your nose. Sniff or inhale cautiously. Do this each time you take your oral nystatin.

If you tolerate this procedure, gradually increase the amount you inhale over the course of several days. Usually 3 or 4 inhalations of nystatin "smoke" will allow the medication to settle on your deeper nasal and sinus membranes.

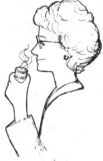

A word of caution: Sometimes your symptoms worsen the first several days you try this procedure. However, stick with it and you may find your symptoms will improve within a few days.

Here's an alternate way of getting nystatin into your upper respiratory passages: Prepare a fresh solution of nystatin, adding 1/16 to 1/8 teaspoon of powder to 4 ounces of boiled and previously cooled water containing 1/4 teaspoon of table salt. Using an ordinary medicine dropper, hold your head back and fill both of your nostrils with the solution. Then swing your head forward rapidly and hold it down between your legs for 2 minutes. Then sit up and let the mixture trickle down your throat.

I haven't yet recommended that patients with yeast-related health problems who have chest symptoms, including bronchitis and asthma, inhale nystatin. And at this time, I would not recommend deep inhalation of nystatin powder unless it was carefully supervised by a physician. Yet, since candida appears to colonize other respiratory membranes, it is possible this type of therapy might help.

Nancy, a 36-year-old factory worker with severe yeast connected problems including fatigue, depression and poor memory, started on a comprehensive treatment program in April, 1983. Her symptoms included extreme fatigue, depression, muscle and joint pain, gastrointestinal symptoms, vaginitis and memory problems. In a followup report on July 1, 1983, Nancy commented,

> "Everything is better, I'm back at work, I've thrown away all my arthritis medicine. And sniffing the nystatin several times a day helps my nasal congestion and memory problems."

Ann, the 30-year-old daughter of Dorothy (see pages 222-223) commented,

> "My nose runs all the time, during every season of the year." Ann was never without a Kleenex® and she usually carried the tissue in her hand. Because Dorothy improved so much on nystatin, she encouraged Ann to try the nystatin nose drops. After using them for a week, Ann's nose cleared. And in a recent phone call she commented, "This is the first time I've enjoyed a dry nose in 20 years."

Your nose may run because of allergies to dozens of things ranging from cat dander to chemicals and from pollens to potatoes. However, if you're troubled by yeast connected health problems and upper respiratory symptoms persist, a trial of intranasal nystatin may help.

11. *Nystatin enemas:* In their article on "Chronic Mucocutaneous Candidiasis," Doctors Charles H. Kirkpatrick and Peter G. Sohnle[44] described candida albicans studies carried out on normal adults by Cohen and associates. The candida organisms were recovered from 30% of the cultures of the mouth and throat, 54% and 55% of various segments of the small intestine, and 65% of the fecal samples. So it would appear that more candida is found in the lower part of the bowel tract than in the upper part.

    Another study by Hofstra[45] and associates (see also page 45) showed that even after large doses of oral nystatin, many stool specimens often contain no measurable amounts of the drug. Accordingly, a nystatin enema would appear to have merit. I particularly recommend nystatin enemas for individuals with severe yeast connected illness, especially those characterized by multiple bowel symptoms, including persistent constipation, who aren't improving using other therapeutic measures.

Here's other data which makes me feel that nystatin enemas are extremely worthwhile even though I've had little experience in using them with my patients:

A. Nystatin acts on intact yeast cells. It binds to components of the yeast cell membranes and, in effect, chisels holes in the membrane. Contents of the yeast cell leak out and the yeast cell dies. So it's obvious that it's important to get the nystatin and the yeast germs together.

B. Over the past decade or more, people who suffer from ulcerative colitis have been helped by cortisone enemas. Cortisone, acting locally on the surfaces of the inflamed membranes, promotes healing and the rectal route has proved quite accessible and has helped countless patients with this disease. Although nystatin and cortisone differ in their therapeutic effects, the goal of getting the medication into the colon where it's most effective is identical.

Before using a nystatin enema, empty your colon using a laxative or cleansing enema. Then add 1/4 to 1/2 teaspoon of nystatin to 8 ounces of salt water (1/2 teaspoon of salt to 8 ounces of water). Retain the enema solution as long as possible.

12. *"Die-off" reactions following nystatin:* When you kill out yeast germs on your intestinal, respiratory or vaginal membranes, you absorb products from these dead yeast germs which temporarily worsen your symptoms. Don't be discouraged. "Stay the course". The more yeast you get rid of, the sooner you'll get better. Many individuals who think that nystatin disagrees with them are experiencing these "die off" reactions. And others who think garlic, onions or cabbage disagree, may be experiencing similar reactions.

Each person is different. When nystatin continues to cause symptoms, including fatigue, depression, aching, feeling "slowed down" and cold, these symptoms can often be relieved by taking a bigger dose of nystatin.

On the other hand, if you're taking 1/2 teaspoon of nystatin and notice that you feel feverish, flushed, stimulated, talkative and other "hyper" symptoms, try taking a smaller dose.

Some patients feel better when they start nystatin, and then weeks later nystatin disagrees. When this happens, the dose should be varied up or down until symptoms are relieved. If adjustment of the nystatin dose continues to present a problem, the efficacy of the nystatin can be enhanced by using garlic, vitamin A and other nutritional supplements, including zinc. Or the carbohydrate content of the diet may temporarily need to be lowered.

13. *Mold control in your home:* Take a look at your house or your workplace. If it's damp and moldy, take measures to reduce the mold content. (See also pages 57-59.)

14. *Lessen your exposure to chemicals:* Make sure you're keeping your chemical exposure at a low level. Perfumes, colognes, cigarette smoke, insecticides, furniture polishes, detergents, gas cooking stoves and other chemical exposures can make you ill . . . especially if your immune system is already weakened by candida (see also pages 151-155).

15. *Try the herbal remedy, taheebo tea:* This substance, also known as Ipe Roxo Herbal Tea and Pau D'Arco or Divine Tree,™ is derived from the inner bark of two South American trees . . . the Lapacho Colorado or Lapacho Marado. These hardwood trees and their leaves apparently contain antifungal substances. Tea from these trees has been used for centuries because of its supposedly curative powers.

A California physician experienced in treating yeast-connected illness commented,

> "Although I know of no studies on the effectiveness of taheebo tea, several of my patients with rather severe yeast problems feel this tea reduces their nystatin requirements. I've been trying it in some of my patients who can't take nystatin and it seems to help."

In commenting further on taheebo tea, she said

> "Several female candida patients are achieving complete alleviation of vaginal yeast symptoms by douching with the same strength of tea as is consumed orally. Douching for several days in a row, then once a week for a few weeks appears to do the trick."

In late July, 1983, I received the following additional information on taheebo tea. A physician with severe chemical sensitivity who had struggled for years to overcome his health problems commented,

> "Drinking a cup of taheebo tea four times a day has played a major role in helping me conquer my yeast-connected illness.
> "The active ingredient in this tea is a substance called *LaPachol* and it's antifungal properties are discussed in an encyclopedia edited by Lewis and Elwin-Lewis."

Moreover, in the National Cancer Institute's *Reports on Plants and Cancer* (Vol. 60, No. 8, August, 1976, pp. 1135-1136), the anticancer properties of LaPachol are discussed."

Early in August 1983, I talked to Paula Davey, M.D., a clinical ecologist from Michigan, who commented, "Clinical expressions from patients show that LaPacho frequently benefits individuals who have been on previous anti-fungal medications and those who have not. The yeast "die off" appears more subtle with the tea than with the nystatin and seems to have a sedative effect on patients. Individual tolerance is variable as it is with any other substance."

During the year 1983, many of my patients tried taheebo tea and some of them reported favorable responses. However, since all of these patients were also using other methods of anti-candida therapy, it has been impossible for me to evaluate the true efficacy of the tea. Moreover, in a phone conversation, Dr. C. Orian Truss told me that studies in his laboratory showed that culture media containing taheebo tea failed to inhibit the growth of candida.

Taheebo and LaPacho tea can be found in many health food stores. Wholesale and retail distributors include I. Fields, 4018 Whittier Blvd., Los Angeles, CA 90023, phone (213) 263-8655, Daniel A. Herman, P.O. Box 5062, So. San Francisco, CA 94083 phone (415) 871-9005, and Priority Products, Inc., 2300 S.E. Belmont St., Portland, OR 97214, phone (503) 239-5949.

16. *Yogurt:* Eating sugar-free yogurt may help you. I recommend this kind of yogurt to all my patients unless they are intolerant or allergic to it. Yogurt contains the friendly germ, *lactobacillus acidophilus,* which helps compete with and control candida in the intestinal tract. In talking to John W. Rippon in December, 1983, he commented,

> "*Lactobacillus acidophilus,* especially if you consume it on a regular basis, restores normal flora to the intestinal tract. I feel it will help patients with yeast-connected health disorders."

(For a further discussion of yogurt see pages 266-267.)

17. *Hormone imbalance:* Many physicians working with yeast-connected illness have found that their patients also suffer from endocrine (hormone) dysfunction which may respond to appropriate therapy prescribed by your physician. In discussing this subject at a conference at Brigham Young University in September, 1982, Dr. Phyllis Saifer said in effect,

"Many patients with environmental illness, including those with yeast-connected problems, appear to have thyroiditis. Yet, the physical examination of the thyroid often shows no irregularities and routine blood studies (T-3, T-4 and TSH) may all be entirely normal. Precise diagnosis is often difficult, although measurement of T-cells may help. I suspect thyroiditis in the difficult to manage brittle patient with symptoms of fatigue, depression, chilling, constipation, irregular menses and other symptoms."

Another physician who has commented on inapparent thyroid disease is Broda Barnes, M.D. In the book *Hypothyroidism: The Unsuspected Illness,* by Broda O. Barnes and Lawrence Galton, Thomas Y. Crowell Company, New York, 1976, the authors comment,

"The normal range of basal temperature is between 97.8° and 98.2° Fahrenheit. When symptoms of thyroid deficiency are present, the basal temperature may be 1 to even 3 degrees below normal. With thyroid therapy, the temperature will start to rise."

Dr. Barnes suggests that patients take a 10-minute axillary (under arm) temperature reading each morning for 7 straight days. If the temperature is consistently under 97.8° to 98.2°, he feels the possibility of thyroid deficiency should be considered and a therapeutic trial of thyroid is recommended. I've tried this technique and therapy in several of my patients and have found that it helped.

Treatment with progesterone may be indicated in patients with premenstrual syndrome (see pages 187, 188) and therapy with estrogen may be indicated in patients with menopausal symptoms.

18. *Treat the marital partner and/or other family members:* Candida, like other microorganisms, can be transmitted from person to person through intimate contact of various sorts including sexual relations. Candida can also be transmitted through nonsexual contacts. Studies by Lucas[4] indicate that candida gets on sheets, pillow cases and clothing and into the air around persons who are colonized with candida.

One of my adult patients with yeast-connected illness commented,

"Going into a basement, cellar or moldy house has always triggered my symptoms and provoked symptoms of fatigue, depression and a 'spaced out' feeling. I noticed the same feelings when I'd pick up my 18-month-old great niece. It got to be embarrassing because I didn't want to pick up the baby. I didn't know why. This was before I learned about yeast. The baby had received many antibiotics and had been troubled by oral thrush and persistent diaper rashes. Now that she's been treated with nystatin and diet, being around her and picking her up doesn't bother me!"

19. *Immunotherapy . . . allergy vaccines:* Many patients with

yeast-related illness are helped by treatment with candida vaccines or extracts (see page 51). Others are helped by appropriate treatment of food and inhalant allergies using allergy extracts. Yet, you may have trouble finding a physician who will use immunotherapy in treating hidden food sensitivities. Here's why:

Allergists resemble people who belong to opposing political parties or who are members of the various religious denominations†. Although most allergists test and treat their patients with allergy extracts, their methods differ considerably. The "traditional" allergists (most of whom are members or Fellows of the American Academy of Allergy and Immunology or the American College of Allergists) usually rely on scratch, prick or RAST tests in evaluating allergic sensitivities in their patients. Most of these allergists use gradually increasing doses of allergy extracts until the maximum tolerated dose is reached. Moreover, allergists of this persuasion rarely use food extracts in treatment. Unquestionably, this "build-up" or high dose method of therapy helps many patients with respiratory allergies caused by inhalants.

However, a growing number of physicians use other methods of testing and treating their patients with yeast, inhalant, food, hormone and chemical sensitivities.[46a,b,c,d,e] Although many of these physicians are members or fellows of the two above mentioned organizations, almost all belong to other allergy societies including the Society for Clinical Ecology, the American Academy of Otolaryngic Allergy and the Pan American Allergy Society.

These allergists generally test their patients with intradermal (within the skin) injections of *serial dilutions* of allergy extracts, as first described by Rinkel,[47] and the *provocative/neutralization techniques* described by Lee and refined by Miller.[46a] The dose of allergy extract used in treatment by these physicians is termed the *optimal* or most effective dose.

During the past 25 years, I've used many different methods of testing and treating my allergic patients and I prefer the Rinkel and Miller methods. Moreover, I've found these methods extremely useful in treating many of my patients who react to so many foods that they experience difficulty in obtaining adequate nutrition.

---

† An 8-page review of the food allergy controversy is presented in the Medical News section of the August 12, 1983 issue of the "Journal of The American Medical Association" (250:701-711, 1983).

Yet, since I became aware of "the yeast connection," I've been treating more and more of my patients with diet, nystatin and nutritional supplements. I've also emphasized the importance of controlling other strands of the "web" of illness-provoking factors. Using such methods, I've found that most of my patients improve and many get well and remain well without allergy testing and immunotherapy. However, other of my patients do not obtain maximum improvement until I test them and give them extracts (administered by injection or sublingually) to help their immune system cope with their inhalant, food and hormone allergies.

Chemical sensitivity presents special problems. Although most of my chemically-sensitive patients improve on diet, nystatin (or other medication), meticulous avoidance of tobacco, perfumes, colognes, formaldehyde, petrochemicals and other volatile chemicals, some individuals are unavoidably exposed to these substances and continue to show troublesome symptoms. I've found that some of these patients are helped, often to a remarkable degree, by provocative testing and neutralization therapy using chemical, formaldehyde and tobacco extracts.

Constance, a registered nurse and the wife of a physician, commented,

"When my children were young I suffered from extreme fatigue and recurrent joint pain. For years I felt bad and it was all I could do to manage. Incidentally, I was fanatical about house cleaning and used aerosol sprays and other odorous cleaners. Yet, I didn't realize that they might be contributing to my problems. I also suffered from persistent nasal drainage. I always had to carry a Kleenex® and every morning I had to clear out my head and chest.

"About 15 years ago, I had a hysterectomy and I felt somewhat better after that, but my respiratory symptoms continued. I would have several rather devastating respiratory infections each year which would take several weeks to clear.

"In the meantime, I'd gradually become aware that chemical fumes and tobacco smoke really bothered me . . . especially tobacco smoke. And if I got in a room where people were smoking, my respiratory symptoms always became worse.

"In 1979 I was tested for tobacco and petrochemicals, and began taking sublingual allergy extracts 2 or 3 times a day. I also began to take extra vitamins and minerals and got rid of a lot of the chemicals in my home. I immediately began to improve, my nose quit running and my postnasal drip almost disappeared. Between 1979 and the spring of 1983, I experienced only one chest infection . . . this was in the late summer of 1980.

"In my work and in my travel, I'm exposed to tobacco smoke, perfumes and other odors; yet with my allergy extracts and extra vitamin C (up to 3,000 or more mgs. a day), I'm able to control my symptoms and stay well most of the time."

20. *Air ionizers:* The air we breathe contains molecules with positive and negative electrical charges. Research studies over a period of several decades show that those who live or work in closed spaces and in environments containing more positive ions than negative ions develop a variety of symptoms. Typical manifestations include fatigue, headache, drowsiness, irritability, nasal discharge, burning eyes and cough. These and other symptoms commonly found in individuals with yeast-connected health disorders may be helped by a negative ion generator. Such generators cost between $75 and $125 and are available from many sources. Further information on the effect of ions can be found in the medical[48a,b] and lay literature[49].

21. *Certain foods kill or inhibit candida:* These include raw garlic, onions, kale, turnips and cabbage. Horseradish and broccoli also inhibit candida growth.

22. *Fruit and grain-induced reactions:* Bananas, oranges, grapes, apples, pears and other fruits may contribute to candida growth, especially if taken in quantity. Fruits are especially apt to produce intestinal gas. If you're eating fruits and aren't doing well, *avoid them.* Then after you improve, you can cautiously try eating small amounts of fruit on a rotated basis (see pages 117-118).

23. *Large doses of vitamin A:* In his book *Candida and Candidosis,*[3] Dr. F. C. Odds points out that independent studies show that mice and rats are less susceptible to candida when given high doses of vitamin A. Yet, vitamin A can be toxic if used in large doses for many months.

Accordingly, when my patients aren't doing well, I usually check their blood vitamin A level. Here's why: Many patients with chronic health problems, especially those involving the gastrointestinal tract, may not absorb nutrients they ingest.

If the vitamin A level is low or borderline low, I prescribe 25,000 International Units daily for a month and then recheck the blood level. An occasional patient will require even larger doses. (Physicians and patients interested in a comprehensive review of vitamin A may wish to consult the article by Donald R. Davis, Ph.D. of the University of Texas entitled, "Using Vitamin A Safely.")[50]

255

24. *Wood burning stoves and fireplaces may aggravate yeast-connected symptoms:* Firewood nearly always contains fungi . . . especially wood cut from dead trees. And logs that are stored often sprout fungi.

25. *Digestive enzymes:* Digestive enzymes, especially Pancreatin, seem to help many of my patients. These enzymes can be purchased without a prescription at most pharmacies and can be taken after each meal and at bedtime. Some patients experience a "die-off" reaction on enzymes the first few weeks they take them.

26. *Clotrimazole:* This synthetic drug became available in the mid-1970's and has been found effective in treating a variety of fungus infections. In one report by Kirkpatrick & Alling[55] troches of clotrimazole were administered 5 times daily to 10 patients with persistent oral candidiasis. These individuals *had not responded to nystatin. Yet they became "completely or nearly asymptomatic in 5 days"* on clotrimzole therapy.

    Clotrimazole creams and suppositories have also been found to be highly effective in treating vaginal candidiasis. However, no data is presently available on the safety and effectiveness of preparations of this drug in reducing candida colonization in the gastrointestinal tract.

27. *Cleaning Foods:* According to James A. O'Shea, M.D., of Lawrence, Massachusetts, foods can be treated in a special bath to remove fungi, insecticide sprays, bacteria and certain chemicals. Here are suggestions adapted and modified from the instructional materials prepared for his patients.

    Treat the fruits and vegetables separately. Use ½ teaspoon of Clorox® to each gallon of water. (Use a stainless steel measuring spoon and do not use products other than the Clorox® brand.)

    Step 1: Place the fresh fruits and/or vegetables into the bath. Soak frozen, leafy vegetables or thin-skin fruits for 15 minutes. Heavy-skin fruits and root vegetables require 20 minutes, a heavy-skin squash 25 minutes. Timing is important. Use a fresh Clorox® bath with each batch of food.

    Step 2: Remove foods from the Clorox® bath and soak them in a clean water bath for 15 minutes. Use fresh, clean water for each batch of food. Once the foods have been cleaned, they are ready for storage in freezer bags.

According to Dr. O'Shea, fruits and vegetables receiving this treatment keep longer, wilted vegetables become crisp and their flavor is enhanced. Most important, mold and chemical contamination is lessened.

28. *Mobilizing your healing resources:* Diet, nystatin, nutritional supplements, avoidance of pollutants and other treatment measures I've talked about play a role in helping you get well. But there are other important areas of healing I've scarcely touched upon. They involve resources available to every human being.

In talking and listening to my patients, I've been repeatedly impressed by those who say, "Faith, hope, and prayer, your caring and your personal interest in me and my problems played an important role in helping me get well."

In his introduction to Norman Cousin's new book, *The Healing Heart*, Bernard Lown, M.D., Professor of Cardiology, Harvard University School of Public Health, pointed out that psychological factors can affect every aspect of human illness. Moreover, Norman Cousins repeatedly documents this relationship in this book as well as in his previous book, *Anatomy of an Illness.* (See also page 166.)

For years I've been putting people on elimination diets for food allergy and watching them get well. In discussing my findings with my old friend, Charles May, M.D., Professor of Pediatrics, Emeritus, of the University of Colorado, Charlie replied,

> "Billy, many of your patients get better because they have faith in you and what you're doing, rather than because of the diets you put them on."

At the time (1976), I disagreed strenuously with Charlie because I knew, beyond any shadow of a doubt, that many, many patients were reacting adversely to foods, including patients who didn't like me and who hated my diets.

But now, as the years have passed, I realize that in some of these patients, at least, improvement was due in part to the interest I took in them as well as to my diets. (I haven't previously admitted this to Charlie!)

As I discussed in an earlier section of this book (page 133-134), countless people enjoy healthy, productive lives because medical science has provided new answers and new therapies. Yet, ever since my internship and residency days, I've been impressed and influenced by caring "people doctors," including my chief at Vanderbilt, Dr.

257

Amos U. Christie, the late Dr. William C. Deamer of the University of California and many others, including physicians in my own state and my own community.

One physician I'll never forget is Dr. F. Tremaine ("Josh") Billings, a Nashville internist. In 1953, my father was hospitalized at Vanderbilt with what proved to be his last illness. Soon after my father arrived in his hospital room about 6:30 on a Sunday evening, Dr. Billings came in to check him. As he sat on the side of the bed and patted my father's arm, my mother commented, "Dr. Jere hasn't eaten anything since lunch and the nurses tell me supper has already been served. . ." Dr. Billings asked, "What does Dr. Jere generally eat for Sunday supper?" My mother replied, "Rice Krispies and bananas with milk and cream."

I've forgotten the exact sequence of events, but Dr. Billings left the room. Then just as the nurse finished taking my father's temperature, Dr. Billings showed up again. A box of Rice Krispies was tucked under one arm, a bottle of milk and cream under the other and in each hand he held a banana. I've never forgotten Dr. Billings' compassion and concern. Certainly he knew, as did the late Francis Peabody, that *"The care of the patient requires caring for the patient."*

So to get well, you'll need to:
   a. Find a caring physician to supervise your overall medical care and, at the same time make sure you aren't suffering from some other organic disease.
   b. Seek also the help of alternative health professionals who are working with patients with yeast-connected health disorders (see also pages 260-264, 267-268).
   c. Locate a lay support group (see page 267). In such a group you'll usually find others who'll share their knowledge with you, provide you with emotional support and help you regain your health. Based on the observations of Norman Cousins, such a support group should encourage laughter, fun, creativity and playfulness. Here's why: Such emotional nutrients mobilize your pain relieving chemicals, the endorphins and help you get well. (See *The Healing Heart*, especially pages 147-158.)

Other Sources of Information

Other sources of information and support on *Candida albicans*, nutrition and on environmental and preventive medicine include:

1. *The Missing Diagnosis,* a 164-page book by C. Orian Truss, M.D. This book, published in early 1983, succinctly describes correctable chronic illnesses associated with chronic candidiasis. Professionals will be especially interested in the three scientific papers of Truss which are reprinted in the Appendix of *The Missing Diagnosis.* For ordering information, write to: *The Missing Diagnosis,* P.O. Box 26508-Y, Birmingham, Alabama 35226.

2. *Update,* a quarterly periodical published by the Gesell Institute of Human Development. Several recent issues of this periodical have discussed the role of *Candida albicans* in causing human illness. Also discussed is the role of nutritional, environmental, psychological and other factors in causing human illness. For further information, send a stamped, self-addressed envelope to: "Update", 310 Prospect Street, New Haven, Connecticut 06511.

3. *Human Ecology Action League (H.E.A.L.).* This national, non-profit organization (with chapters in many cities) publishes a quarterly magazine, "The Human Ecologist". This periodical contains news on recent developments in environmental medicine, including sources of books, food, clothing and other supplies. Beginning in 1980, a number of issues have discussed the relationship of *Candida albicans* to the health problems of the chemically-sensitive individual. For information about the newsletter or a support group in your area send a stamped, self-addressed envelope to: "H.E.A.L.", P.O. Box 1369, Evanston, Illinois 60611.

4. *The Price-Pottenger Nutrition Foundation,* a non-profit, educational foundation, incorporated in the State of California, publishes a quarterly bulletin devoted to various nutritional topics, including the relationship of *Candida albicans* to human illness. For further information send a stamped, self-addressed envelope to: PPNF, P.O. Box 2614, La Mesa, California 92041.

5. *The Journal of Orthomolecular Psychiatry,* publication office, 2229 Broad Street, Regina Saskatchewan, Canada S4P 1Y7. This journal, published in Canada, provides information on a wide variety of topics including *Candida albicans,* vitamins, trace minerals and other subjects relevant to lay persons as well as professionals.

6. The *People's Medical Society,* 33 E. Minor Street, Emmaus, PA. This organization is the project of the Soil and Health Society, a non-profit, tax exempt organization. It was organized to create a national citizen's group to promote preventive health practices and contain medical costs. Services include a regular newsletter. Membership fee is $20 per year.

7. *The National Women's Health Network,* 224 7th Street, SE, Washington, D.C. 20003. This organization is the "nation's only consumer organization devoted to women's health issues." Members have access to a large resource library and are sent information on request. They also receive a bi-monthly newsletter on the latest health information. Membership fees are $25 per year for individuals and $30 per year for groups.

8. *The Environmental Health Association of Dallas, Inc.,* P. O. Box 224121, Dallas, TX 75264, provides information and support to individuals with chronic health disorders including illness related to *Candida albicans.* They publish a newsletter, *Twentieth Century Living.* For further information, send them a self-addressed, stamped envelope.

9. *The Center for Science in the Public Interest (CSPI),* provides a variety of excellent materials on nutrition. Their monthly 16-page publication, *Nutrition Action,* is well written, interesting and authoritative. For further information send a stamped, self-addressed envelope to: CSPI, 1775 S Street, Washington, D.C. 20009.

10. *Western New York (WNY) Allergy and Ecology Association* (Secretary, Rika VanderWalt, 437 Linwood Avenue, Buffalo, NY 14209.) Available through this organization is a newsletter which reviews relevant literature and contains general information for individuals with food and chemical sensitivity and yeast-connected health disorders. Price for 10 issues per year is $10. Single issue—$1.

11. *Nutrition for Optimal Health Association (NOHA).* Available from this non-profit organization are educational materials, including tapes, books and a newsletter. For further information send a stamped, self-addressed envelope to: NOHA, P.O. Box 380, Winnetka, Illinois 60093.

12. *Allergy Management and Support Group* c/o Mrs. Judy Hall,

4356 Sadalia, Toledo, Ohio, 43623. Phone (419) 885-4019.

13. *Allergy Information Association (A.I.A.) of Canada,* Room 7, 25 Poynter Drive, Weston, Ontario M9R 1KB. This organization founded in 1964 publishes an excellent quarterly newsletter *Allergy Shot* which provides information on allergies and a wide variety of related health topics.

14. *Access to Nutritional Data,* P. O. Box 52, Ashby, Massachussetts 01431, (617) 386-7002. Information about nutrition is exploding and almost impossible to keep up with. This organization publishes monthly file cards summarizing the nutritional literature. Subscription rates are $80 for six months, $150 for 12 months.

15. *Insta-Tape, Inc.,* 810 South Myrtle Avenue, P. O. Box 1729, Monrovia, California 91016. This company provides educational tapes for professionals and nonprofessionals dealing with a variety of topics relating to allergy, clinical ecology and nutrition.

16. *Action Against Allergy,* 43 The Downs, London, England SW20 8HG. (A registered charitable company limited by guarantee.) This association is working to help people with chronic illness related to foods, chemicals and yeasts. Chairperson: Mrs. Amelia Nathan Hill.

17. *Allergy Alert.* A monthly newsletter by Sally Rockwell discussing food, chemical and other allergies and yeast-connected health disorders. For further information send a self-addressed, stamped envelope to *Allergy Alert,* P. O. Box 15181, Seattle, Washington 98115. Also available from this source is *Rotation Game,* "a self-help survival kit for those with food allergies and a handbook of recipes entitled *Coping With Candida.*"

18. *Sara Sloan Nutra,* P. O. Box 13825, Atlanta, GA 30324. Available from this source is a nutrition newsletter and a variety of helpful books and pamphlets directed especially toward improving the nutritional status of children.

19. *Metabolic Update.* A monthly audio tapes service designed to alert the listner to fast breaking advances in nutrition by Jeffery Bland, Ph.D., of the Linus Pauling Institute. $150 per year, $20 per copy. For information write Jeffrey Bland's *Metabolic Update,* 15615 Bellevue-Redmond Road, Suite E, Bellevue, WA 98008.

20. *Health Guidance Center*, 18975 Villa View Road, Cleveland, OH 44119, (216) 486-6888. This non-profit center was organized to disseminate information about nutrition, preventive health and illness related to *Candida albicans*.

21. *Brain/Mind Bulletin*, Box 4221, Los Angeles, California 90042. This newsletter (edited by Marilyn Ferguson, author of *The Aquarian Conspiracy*) deals with medicine, psychology, learning and related subjects. $20 per year

22. *Human Ecology Foundation of Canada*, (medical advisor John G. Maclennan, M.D.), 465 No. 8 Highway, Dundas, Ontario L9H 4V9. This foundation publishes a quarterly newsletter. It was organized to provide information for those interested in obtaining safe sources of food, clothing and housing. Annual membership fee is $20.

23. *Executive Health*. This 6 to 8 page highly authoritative publication discusses dozens of topics you need to know about if you want to take charge of your health and stay well (see also pages 246, 298). Published monthly by Executive Health Publications, P. O. Box 589, Rancho Santa Fe, California 92067. Subscriptions are $30 per year in U.S.A., Canada, and Mexico.

24. *Huxley Institute for Biosocial Research (HIBR)*, 219 East 31st Street, New York, New York 10016. This non-profit national organization carries on a number of educational activities. Included are training seminars for physicians and yearly symposia for the public. Their goals include providing both professionals and non-professionals with the latest findings in nutrition and more especially in orthomolecular medicine and psychiatry.

25. *Canadian Schizophrenia Foundation*, 2229 Broad Street, Regina, Saskatchewan, S4P 1Y7, Canada. This is the Canadian "sister organization" of the Huxley Institute. Its goals and purposes are identical. Certain classes of membership in either of these organizations include subscriptions to the quarterly *Journal of Orthomolecular Psychiatry* and a quarterly newsletter.

26. *Schizophrenia Association of Greater Washington (SAGW)*, Wheaton Place Office Building, North, #404, Wheaton, Maryland 20902. This organization was founded primarily to help individuals with schizophrenia, depression and other mental illnesses. However, it now also serves as a resource organization for both professionals and non-professionals interested

in alternative approaches to health care.

27. *The International Journal of Biosocial Research*, P. O. Box 1174, Tacoma, Washington 98401. This quarterly publication "is a peer-review inter-disciplinary journal devoted to research on the environmental, genetic, biochemical and nutritional factors affecting human behavior and social groupings."

28. En-Trophy Institute, Box 984, Station "A", Hamilton, Ontario L8N 3R1, Canada. This organization publishes the *En-Trophy Review*, a "unique" wholistic approach to your food and health.

29. *The People's Doctor*, an informative, stimulating and provocative newsletter by Robert Mendelsohn, M.D., an articulate advocate of preventive health and alternative methods of health care. For more information, write to *The People's Doctor*, P. O. Box 982, Evanston, IL 60204.

30. *The Preventive Medicine Doctor*, by M. J. Packovich, M.D. This pamphlet (published by TECBOOK PUBLICATIONS, P. O. Box 5002, Topeka, KS 66605 - price $1.39) lists the names and addresses of 140 publications and 121 associations, including both orthodox and alternative health care approaches. Many of these offer newsletters, booklets and magazines for low cost or without charge.

31. *Kup's Komments*. A Holistic Journal for patients, public and health practitioners, by Roy Kupsinel, M.D., P. O. Box 550, Oviedo, Florida 32765.

32. *Once Daily*, by Jerome Mittleman, D.D.S. "A new digest of dental health for people who want sound teeth and healthy bodies." 263 West End Ave., #2-A, New York, N.Y. 10023.

33. *Yeast Tapes*. I learn something new about yeast-connected illness almost every day. Sometimes such information comes from another physician. Yet, astute observations also come from my patients. Conferences I attend and articles in either the medical or lay literature also help.

To pass along some of this information, I'm preparing a series of audio tapes. For further information, send a stamped, self-addressed envelope to: *Yeast Information*, Box 1000, Jackson, Tennessee 38301.

British Sources of Help and Information

1. *Action Against Allergy*, 43 The Downs, London, England SW20 8HG.
2. *The McCarrison Society*, Miss Pauline Atkin, Secretary, 23 Stanley Court, Worcester Road, Sutton, Surrey SM2 65D, England.
3. *Hyperactive Children's Support Group*, 59 Meadowside, Angmering, West Sussex, England.
4. *Sanity*, 77 Moss Lane, Pinner, Middlesex, England HA5 3A0.
5. *Schizophrenia Association of Great Britain*, Tyr Twr, Ooanfair Hall, Caernarvon, Wales OL55 1TT.
6. *The Journal of Alternative Medicine*, 30 Station Approach, West Byfleet, Surrey, England KT14 GNF.
7. *Clinical Ecology Society*, The Medical Center, Michael J. Radcliffe, M.D., President, Hythe, Southampton, England S04 52B.

37

What You Can Do If Your Physician Is Unaware Of The Yeast Connection

If your health complaints are yeast-connected, you may experience diffi-culty in finding a physician to help you. Here's why: The three pub-lished articles[51abc] by C. Orian Truss on *Candida albicans* and its relationship to human illness aren't available in most medical li-braries. Accordingly, most physicians haven't had an opportunity to read them. And even if a physician has heard of "the yeast con-nection" he may say, "There's no proof that candida plays a role in making you sick." Or "Where are the scientific studies?"

If you read medical history (or even if you take a look at medical practice today) you'll find that acceptance of new ideas and infor-mation has always been slow. It takes time for it to filter down through the ranks. Moreover, Jim Johnson, a Chicago physician, recently commented that people often do not want to learn what they don't already know. Jim Willoughby, a Kansas City physi-cian, has similarly noted that if a physician isn't "up" on a subject he tends to be "down" on it.

If your physician isn't aware of the role candida may be playing in human illness here are things you can do:

(1) Lend or give your physician your copy of *The Yeast Connec-tion;*

(2) Order Dr. Truss' book, *The Missing Diagnosis,* and read it. Then lend or give it to your physician. This book contains the three original Truss articles plus much additional information (book price $27.50 postpaid). Order from *The Missing Diagnosis,* P.O. Box 26508, Birmingham, AL 35226.

(3) Send a stamped, self-addressed envelope to the Price-

Pottenger Foundation, P.O. Box 2614, La Mesa, California 92041. This organization keeps a roster of physicians interested and knowledgeable in treating yeast-connected health problems.

(4) Even without the help of a physician (to prescribe nystatin or other medication) you can make changes in your diet and lifestyle which will strengthen your immune system and reduce the load of yeasts in your body. Here are suggestions:

A. Study the diet instructions (pages 73-110.) If your symptoms are mild, start with the *Candida Control Diet* (pages 73-84). If they're severe begin with the Low Carbohydrate Diet (pages 94-110), or the Fruit-Free, Sugar-Free Diet (pages 117-120). If you improve in a week or two after making these dietary changes, you can experiment and "cheat" occasionally and see which foods trigger your symptoms . . .

B. Rotate your diet. Food intolerances or allergies are more apt to bother people who eat the same foods every day, especially if they eat them several times a day.

C. *Supplement your diet with the friendly bacteria, Lactobacillus acidophilus* (L.A.) Here's information on such supplementation obtained in an article† by George Von Hilsheimer, Ph.D.

> "Observations of a long series of psychiatric patients disclosed a deficiency of *Lactobacillus acidophilus* (L.A.) in their stools associated with GI symptoms and other evidences of idiosyncratic responses to food. . .
>
> "Supplementation with high levels of L.A. in the form of freeze dried L.A. in capsules, L.A. cultured milk yogurt or L.A. implanted milk ("sweet acidophilus") resulted in grossly observable changes in stool, increase in stool L.A. and reduction of symptoms associated with food.

In discussing L.A. supplementation Dr. Von Hilsheimer pointed out that Professor Marvin L. Speck and his associates in the Department of Food Science, North Carolina State University, Raleigh, North Carolina, in 1977, found that commercial products advertising L.A. content in conjunction with other lactobacilli in fact do *not* contain appreciable numbers of "L.A.".

In a letter to me on February 2, 1984 Dr. Von Hilsheimer sent me these instructions for making yogurt:

---

†Von Hilsheimer, G.L. Acidophilus and the Ecology of the Human Gut. *Journal of Orthomolecular Psychiatry 11:3, 204-207, 1982.*

"Use acidophilus milk from the supermarket. Fill only one of the cups of a standard yogurt maker and leave the yogurt maker on with milk in it from the carton. Do not preheat or scald the milk!!! Usually this will separate into curds and whey. Discard the whey (or use it in soup). Use the thick white curd as yogurt starter. Follow directions with your yogurt maker, but use a regular milk for the yogurt and not your acidophilus milk.

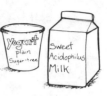

1. Take out the yogurt maker.
2. Pour a cup of acidophilus milk, without processing it in any way, directly from the carton into one of the yogurt making cups.
3. Turn the maker on and leave it 8-12 hours
4. Use the white thick material which is produced for starter just as if it was yogurt, or commercial starter.
5. Use regular milk and follow the directions with your yogurt maker.

Some lucky people seem regularly to be able to make the yogurt directly from acidophilus milk by watching closely and stopping the process. If you are one of those born-again cooks you can short circuit the process. But after advising hundreds of patients I find that most people get better results by following steps 1-5 above."

D. Supplement your diet with yeast-free vitamin-mineral preparations. Such supplementation should include zinc, calcium, magnesium, Vitamins A, B complex (yeast-free), C and selenium. Garlic may also help combat candida (see discussion on page 291-292).

E. Supplement your diet with essential fatty acids which are especially rich in important nutrients your body needs: (1.) Linseed oil — one-half to two tablespoons daily. This oil can be mixed with lemon juice and used as a salad dressing. (2.) Evening primrose oil — one or two capsules two or three times a day.

F. Lighten the load of pollutants in your home or work place. (See pages 139-140 and 151-162).

G. Exercise regularly.
H. Stop smoking. Avoid birth control pills and antibiotics (where possible).
I. Put your "emotional house" in order. Love, touch, faith, hope and prayer are all important in helping you get well and stay well.

If you're tired, discouraged, sick and depressed you may find it difficult to follow the above program without help and support. Fortunately, many alternative health care facilities and groups are being developed throughout the United States, Canada and England. In the December 15, 1983 issue of the *New England Journal of Medicine* (309:1524-1527, 1983), John Lister, M.D., Farm End., Burkes Road, Beaconsfield, HP9 IPB England, in a commentary entitled, *Current Controversy On Alternative Medicine*, had this to say:

> "For various reasons there seems to be an increasing dissatisfaction with certain aspects of conventional or orthodox medicine." " . . . one of the growth industries in contemporary Britain is — *alternative medicine.*"

Dr. Lister told of the formation of the British Holistic Medicine Association and of the growing debate in England, especially since the London Times published three major articles on various aspects of alternative medicine as well as an editorial entitled, "Physician Heal Thyself".

In its editorial the Times supported the concept of alternative medicine and was highly critical of those who resist alternative approaches to health care, and further stated,

> "There is a growing loss of faith by the public in a purely scientific approach to medicine.
> Moreover, such an open approach seems to present the British National Health Service with an insatiable demand for all kinds of surgery and with a drug bill for billions of pounds with its inevitable component of dangerous mistakes. It is recognized that orthodox medicine has great scientific achievements to its credit but the Times believes that it is ungenerous in its attitude to alternative systems or treatment when scientific research has failed to provide satisfactory answers.

In his article, Dr. Lister also presented the ideas of those who defend contemporary methods of medical practice. Yet, he noted,

"There is often an arrogant reluctance of the medical profession to accept—or even to consider—healing methods which haven't been confirmed by scientific studies."

In concluding his commentary, Dr. Lister emphasizes that the physician's "first priority" must be to make sure that he or she is not missing treatable organic diseases, especially in patients with rather vague symptoms. Having done so, he or she may then use whatever methods "are available and appropriate" and that "if such methods are unorthodox they should be considered as *complementary* rather than *alternative* to orthodox methods (see also pages 258-264). Nearly all emphasize better nutrition, exercise and lifestyle changes rather than relying on prescription drugs and surgery.

In his recent book, *(The Healing Heart)*, Norman Cousins expresses similar thoughts in a chapter entitled "Consumerism Reaches Medicine:"

"Holistic medicine is an expression of, not a substitute for, the best in traditional medical practice . . . The new consumerism need not be regarded as a threat to medicine or as anything alien."

The rise of consumerism and the growing interest in alternative health care was also discussed recently by Marilyn Ferguson:

"One major arena, health care, has already begun to experience wrenching change . . . For all its reputed conservatism, western medicine is undergoing an amazing revitalization. Patients and professionals alike are beginning to see beyond symptoms to the context of illness. stress, society, family, diet, season, emotions . . . Hospitals, long the bastions of barren efficiency, are scurrying to provide more humane environments for birth and death . . .

"A guest editorial in *American Medical News* decried medicine's crisis of human relations . . . 'Physicians must recognize that medicine is not their private preserve but a profession in which all people have a vital stake'."†

In her continuing discussion, Ms. Ferguson referred to the influence of Norman Cousins and pointed out that informal discussion groups on holistic approaches to medicine were meeting regularly

†Excerpted from *The Aquarian Conspiracy; Personal and Social Transformation in the 1980s*, ©1980 by Marilyn Ferguson. Published by J.P. Tarcher, Inc., 9110 Sunset Blvd., Los Angeles, CA 90069. $15.00, $8.95 soft cover. Used by permission.

at such medical schools as UCLA, University of Texas in Galveston, Baylor in Houston and Johns Hopkins in Baltimore. And in her concluding remarks in her chapter on health, she said:

> "Surely, historians will marvel at the heresy we fell into, the recent decades in which we disregarded the spirit in our efforts to cure the body. Now, in finding health, we find ourselves."

Here's more: John Naisbitt, in his current bestseller, *Megatrends — Ten New Directions Transforming Our Lives*†, noted the growing interest in health promoting diets, exercise and self care. And he commented on several major trends in health, including:

> "The triumph of the new paradigm of wellness, preventive medicine and wholistic care over the old model of illness, drugs, surgery and treating symptoms rather than the whole person."

I've heard it said, "There's nothing more powerful than an idea whose time has come." So when you take charge of your life and health, you'll be joining millions of other folks all over America.

---

†*Megatrends — Ten New Directions Transforming Our Lives,* 1982 by John Naisbitt. Published by Warner Books, 666 5th Avenue, New York, NY 10103.

38
Summary Of The 1982 Dallas Informal Conference

According to Odds[3], hundreds of articles appear each year on Candida albicans. Yet, until the three articles by Truss published in the *Journal of Orthomolecular Psychiatry*[51 a,b,c] beginning in 1978 (followed by the Truss Book[2] in 1983), few, if any, reports in the medical literature discussed the type of yeast-connected illnesses which are the subject of this book. And even today . . . summer, 1983 . . . only scant additional medical references are available to help physicians seeking further information.

Yet, during the years, 1981-1983, interest in the relationship of Candida albicans to human illness has skyrocketed. This interest has also been stimulated by discussions on TV† and radio and in magazines and newspapers.

In spite of this tremendous demand from the public for more information, additional reports on immune system disorders related to *Candida albicans* in the medical literature have been limited to one article[1] and several Letters to the Editor[20 ''], Accordingly, I felt it appropriate to briefly summarize the discussions of the Informal Conference on Candida Albicans and the Relationship to Human Disease held in Dallas, Texas, July 9, 10 and 11, 1982.

Some 20 physicians who had been working with patients with candida-related illness during the years 1979-1982 met and presented

---

† Dr. Truss and one of his patients, Suzi Elman, were interviewed by Sandi Freeman on *Freeman Reports* (Cable News Network) in September, 1981. According to Sandi, "This program brought more mail and phone calls than any previous program."

I discussed yeast-connected health problems with Bob Braun (Braun and Company, WLW-TV, Cincinnati) in January, 1983. Within 7-days, my office received 7,300 requests for more information.

271

their experiences informally. An additional 20 to 30 physicians participated in the general discussion. Several physicians commented,

"I have more questions than answers."

Most participants agreed that *the history was the most useful tool in diagnosing candida-related illness.* And many physicians emphasized the role of prolonged antibiotic use in contributing to the development of this illness.

Nearly all participants agreed that symptoms referable to the nervous system, the reproductive organs (especially in adult females) and the gastrointestinal systems were especially prominent. However, involvement of every body system was reported. And individuals of all ages and both sexes can be affected.

All physicians used nystatin in treating patients with candida-related illness. However, experiences were varied in regard to the most effective dose. Several participants described nystatin reactions, including fatigue, depression and nausea. There was considerable discussion as to the mechanism of these reactions. The predominant feeling was that reactions were caused by yeast "die-off", caused by toxins released from killed candida organisms.

Experiences with diet were also varied. Some participants felt that an initial low carbohydrate diet (60 to 80 grams) was essential to obtain improvement. Other participants felt that complex or "good" carbohydrates (vegetables, whole grains and fruits) could be eaten and that only sugar and other refined carbohydrates need be restricted (unless a person was allergic to a particular food such as wheat or corn). All participants emphasized the importance of foods with high mold content and environmental molds in triggering symptoms.†

---

† Many other yeasts and molds are closely related to *Candida albicans* including *Trichophyton* and *Epidermophyton.* A number of physicians treating yeast-connected health problems (including Lawrence Dickey, M.D., of Fort Collins, Colorado) have found that immunotherapy using an extract containing these two molds plus candida is often more effective than nystatin therapy or than candida extract alone. (The combined extract containing the three yeasts and molds is often termed "TCE", "TOE", or "TME").

Recently Walter Ward, M.D., an otolaryngologist and allergist of Winston-Salem, North Carolina, commented, "I'm using a great deal of anti-fungal therapy including nystatin, Nizoral® and immunotherapy and getting fantastic results." Dr. Ward also reported that extracts from the mold *Microsporum* helped some of his patients with yeast-connected illness who hadn't been completely relieved by other therapies. Among these patients were several individuals with skin problems, including psoriasis.

Experiences in using immunotherapy were varied. Several physicians told of successful use of extremely minute dilutions of candida extract . . . dilutions that were "homeopathic" in nature with one part candida to one-quadrillion or one-quintillion parts of diluting fluid; others recommended more potent doses of candida extract, based on provocative testing and neutralization. No participants recommended the traditional "build-up" method of immunotherapy with candida extracts.

All agreed that candida extracts, when used, required careful and repeated monitoring by the physician, and that no automatic protocol for use of such extracts could be provided for the physician or patient.

In discussing nystatin . . .

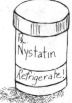

a. The great majority of the conference participants felt that it was an unusually safe medicine which has been given to thousands of patients over a period of many years without serious adverse reactions.

b. Most participants agreed that in patients with the typical history which suggests yeast-connected illness, a therapeutic trial of nystatin and diet should be continued for 2 to 3 months before "giving up" and deciding that a patient's illness had no relation to Candida albicans.

c. Concerning the duration of nystatin therapy in patients who were responding to an anti-candida treatment program, most physicians reported that they found they could gradually discontinue nystatin in 6 to 12 months as the patient's immune system and health improved. However, some patients required nystatin for several years before their recovery was complete.

There was considerable discussion of patients with chemical sensitivity. Such patients have been found to show impairment of the immune system (including reduction of T cells) in a manner similar to patients with yeast-connected health problems. Several observers told of patients who had been chemical victims with severe and continuing chemical sensitivity who recovered following anti-candida treatment.

A number of physicians emphasized the importance of a comprehensive program of management. Their therapeutic approach included not only anti-candida therapy, but also the avoidance and appropriate management of hidden food and chemical allergies. In managing such allergies, they found that provocative testing and immunotherapy with food and chemical extracts were highly effective.

Many participants noted a close relationship between the immune, endocrine and nervous systems. And hormonal imbalances in female patients often appeared to be triggered by candida-related illness. Moreover, when candida and the accompanying immune system disorder was appropriately treated, hormonal problems often improved, sometimes dramatically.

A few physicians reported dramatic results in treating patients with severe and often "incurable" auto-immune diseases, including multiple sclerosis, Crohn's disease, arthritis and schizophrenia. And several physicians told of the favorable results using an anti-candida program in treating severe and disabling chronic skin disorders, including psoriasis.

Many participants emphasized that candida-related illness was not "a disease" and that many different factors played a role in causing people to be ill. Included among these factors are not only candida, but also nutritional deficiencies, allergies and psychological deprivation or trauma.

The entire Dallas Conference was recorded. Physicians and other professionals (and non-professionals, too) can obtain cassette tapes (12 hours of recording) from Creative Audio, 8751 Osborne, Highland, Indiana 46322, price $58.00.

A second conference, *The Yeast-Human Interaction, 1983*, was held in Birmingham, Alabama on December 9-11, 1983. This symposium was organized "to exchange ideas about the chemistry, immunology, microbiology, diagnosis and therapy of imbalances in the relationship between humans and the yeasts . . . of their flora, food and environment." It was sponsored by the Gesell Institute of Human Development, New Haven, Connecticut, and the Critical Illness Research Foundation, Inc. Birmingham, Alabama.

The faculty consisted of the following:

Sidney MacDonald Baker, M.D.
   New Haven, Connecticut
Eunice Carlson, Ph. D.
   Houghton, Michigan
Max D. Cooper, M.D.
   Birmingham, Alabama
William G. Crook, M.D.
   Jackson, Tennessee

Leo Galland, M.D.
  New Haven, Connecticut
Kazuo Iwata, M.D.
  Tokyo, Japan
Alan S. Levin, M.D.
  San Francisco, California
Warren R. Pistey, M.D., Ph.D.
  Bridgeport, Connecticut
John W. Rippon, Ph.D.
  Chicago, Illinois
E. William Rosenberg, M.D.
  Memphis, Tennessee
C. Orian Truss, M.D.
  Birmingham, Alabama
Francis J. Waickman, M.D.
  Cuyahoga Falls, Ohio

The entire proceedings of the conference were professionally recorded by Creative Audio, 8751 Osborne, Highland, IN 46322. The price for the 20 hours of recording is $118. Video tapes are also available.

39

Potpourri

It seems that almost every day I learn things about yeast-connected illness I didn't know before. This chapter includes information I've acquired from various sources in the past year or two, especially during the fall and winter of 1983-84. Although some of this material is directed mainly to physicians, it should interest anyone with a health problem related to *Candida albicans*.

Observations of Practicing Physicians:† In October, 1983 I mailed a 27 item questionnaire to a number of physicians, each of whom had treated hundreds of patients with yeast-connected health disorders. Here's a summary of their observations:

* Each patient is unique and different and no program of therapy fits every patient.
* While anti-candida therapy featuring diet and nystatin is important, all patients require comprehensive management.
* Most of the clinicians emphasized the importance of the low carbohydrate diet. However, most felt that complex carbohydrates should be gradually returned to the diet as the patient improves.
* Several physicians suggested placing patients on the "Cave Man", "Stone Age" or Low Carbohydrate Diet for one week before beginning nystatin. In this way yeasts were "starved out" and die-off reactions from the nystatin were less troublesome.
* Success was reported in using initial doses of nystatin of one

---

†Doctors Jim Brodsky of Chevy Chase, Maryland; John Curlin of Jackson, Tennessee; Lawrence Dickey of Fort Collins, Colorado; Ken Gerdes of Denver, Colorado; Howard Hagglund of Norman, Oklahoma; Harold Hedges of Little Rock, Arkansas; George Kroker of La Crosse, Wisconsin; Don Lewis of Jackson, Tennessee; Allan Lieberman of North Charleston, South Carolina; Richard Mabray of Victoria, Texas; George Mitchell of Washington, D.C.; Gary Oberg of Crystal Lake, Illinois; James O'Shea of Lawrence, Massachusetts; Phyllis Saifer of Berkeley, California; and Morton Teich of New York, New York.

million units (1/4th teaspoon of powder or two tablets) four times a day rather than smaller doses of 500,000 units (1/8th teaspoon of powder or 1 tablet) or "dot doses" of powder.

- Several physicians mentioned their successful use of ketoconazole (Nizoral®) in treating many of their patients, especially those who did not respond to nystatin. One physician recommended giving Nizoral® in a dose of two tablets daily for the first week of therapy to bring the patient's symptoms under control. As the patient improved, nystatin was often added to the treatment program. The dose of Nizoral® could then usually be reduced or discontinued. No serious toxic reactions were noted from Nizoral® use. (See also pages 48-49)
- Nearly all physicians used nutritional supplements including vitamin C in doses of 1,000 milligrams (or more) routinely. Larger doses of vitamin C were administered to patients with fever or following chemical exposure or under stress. The "bowel tolerance test" was suggested as a method of determining the proper dose (see pages 244-245).
- Nearly all physicians used immunotherapy with candida extracts or candida extracts combined with 2 other molds, trichophyton and epidermophyton ("TCE" or TOE"). Most physicians used relatively stronger dilutions of vaccine.
- Most physicians also used immunotherapy for inhalants, foods and chemicals. However, several felt that such immunotherapy was less often necessary in patients who followed a comprehensive anti-candida treatment program including diet, nystatin and/or Nizoral®.

All but two of the physicians who responded to the questionnaire practice allergy and clinical ecology. Each was asked to make a statement as to how anti-candida therapy had influenced or changed his/her practice. Here are representative responses:

"Makes most other forms of treatment (except some relatively uncomplicated food avoidance) unnecessary in most cases."

"Anticandida therapy is *only a part of my regular treatment program.* Major foods and chemicals are just as important."

"I now regard anticandida therapy as "the most indispensable tool." Though in selected patients, chemicals and foods are equally important. I'd hate to do without either."

"Anticandida treatment is primary in 75-80 percent of my patients. Such therapy helps in a lot of patients who would have been marginally functional with food and chemical avoidance."

"I feel that anticandida therapy has revolutionized my practice in allergy and clinical ecology. I feel it is a "cornerstone" in the treatment of many chronic health problems in children."

"*I'm becoming a yeastologist.* Most patients in my practice seem to have the yeast problem. However, no one program will fit all yeast-affected patients. It is a highly individualized problem which varies from patient to patient."

"Anti-yeast therapy has dramatically helped my patients and changed my practice. Yeast control should be tried in all ecologically ill patients."

"Because of my emphasis on candida, I've attracted a large number of candida patients. Approximately 50% of the patients in my practice require anticandida therapy."

"I believe anticandida therapy is appropriate in virtually 100% of allergy and clinical ecology patients. This confirms my previous findings that seasonal gynecological problems were more often correlated with molds spore counts than with pollen counts."

"50% of my patients have some kind of yeast problem. In 10% it may be the entire problem."

"Anticandida therapy has changed my approach to patients dramatically. 75% of my practice is on anticandida therapy."

Amphotericin B: A special report to physicians.† According to the Physician's Desk Reference (1983 edition) "This antibiotic, first isolated . . . by the Squibb Institute for Medical Research, *is substantially more active in vitro against candida strains than nystatin,* and has been widely used by the intravenous route in the treatment of many deep-seated mycotic infections. Given orally amphotericin B *is extremely well tolerated and is virtually nontoxic in prophylactic doses.* Although poorly absorbed from the gut, amphotericin B has a high degree of activity against candida species in the intestinal tract . . . ."

Yet in spite of this effectiveness and safety when given orally, such preparations of amphotericin B aren't available in the United States except in combination with tetracycline.†† Accordingly, I hadn't thought of using oral amphotericin B in treating my patients. Then in January, 1983 a physician with severe chemical sensitivity and other yeast-connected immune system problems commented,

"I've been taking oral amphotericin B and it has changed my life. I suffered from severe health problems for years and had to live like a

†See also footnote on page 260.
††Mysteclin-F® (Squibb)

hermit. When I began sticking to my yeast-free, low-carbohydrate diet and taking nystatin, I improved significantly. Yet, chemical exposures still bothered me and I was afraid to go into public places.

"In early 1983 I became interested in oral amphotericin B and through a friend in Paris I filled a prescription for Fungizone® (the Squibb name for amphotericin B marketed in France). I've been taking 250 mg. of this drug 2 or 3 times a day for the past couple of months and have improved even more than had been possible on nystatin."

In his continuing discussion this physician commented,

"I also sniff or inhale the amphotericin powder — so it reaches the candida on my nasal and sinus membranes. This relieves my nasal symptoms and lessens my fatigue and headache. *It really is effective.*"

After receiving this anecdotal report I began to look for more information about amphotericin B. I talked to the director of the Cancer Research Program at an eastern university who commented,

"We have recently been using oral amphotericin B in special situations and are now treating 21 patients with this drug." In commenting further he said, "I wish oral amphotericin B (without tetracycline) was available in this country. Yet it seems there hasn't been enough demand for such preparations to make it economically feasible for Squibb to market them in the United States."

In investigating further the efficacy and safety of oral amphotericin B, I found a fascinating report in the medical literature by Montes, Cooper & associates of the University of Alabama (*Prolonged Oral Treatment of Chronic Mucocutaneous Candidiasis with Amphotericin B:* Arc. Derm. 104:45-55, 1971). These investigators gave this drug orally to four patients with chronic mucocutaneous candidiasis using a total daily dose of 1,000 to 1,800 milligrams for six to fourteen months. "In all four patients oral administration of amphotericin B was free of side affects. *Likewise frequent laboratory studies failed to show abnormalities.*"

Montes, Cooper & associates also described studies of other investigators who had used amphotericin B in daily doses of 1000 mgs. or more for many months in treating systemic fungal infections. In discussing the possible toxicity of the drug, these investigators commented,

"In the studies† just mentioned, as well as in our own patients, amphotericin B tablets given orally showed a remarkable lack of clinical and laboratory toxicity."

In their concluding comments, these authors stated:

"It would seem parodoxical at a time when the usefulness of antibiotic combinations has been seriously questioned that amphotericin B tablets can be prescribed in combined form designed to prevent candidiasis but cannot be obtained to be used alone to treat candidiasis."

Because of the well-known toxicity of intravenous amphotericin B, I continued to search for further information about the oral use of this drug. According to Goodman and Gilman's Pharmacological Basis of Therapeutics (6th Ed., 1980, pgs. 1233-1236), amphotericin B, like nystatin, is a polyene antibiotic whose mechanism of action in destroying candida organisms is identical to that of nystatin. Like nystatin, amphotericin B is poorly absorbed from the intestinal tract.

Moreover, even in doses three times greater than those used by Montes, Cooper & associates, plasma levels of amphotericin B were only one-third to one-fifteenth as great as those reached on intravenous administration. These data certainly suggest that oral amphotericin B should be a safe alternative anti-candida medication — especially for patients who: (1) do not tolerate nystatin, (2) fail to improve on nystatin or (3) relapse while taking nystatin after an initial period of improvement.

Between March and August of 1983, a number of my patients who did not tolerate nystatin or who failed to improve while taking nystatin obtained amphotericin B from France and several showed an excellent response.

Laura, a 39-year-old teacher, had been troubled by headaches and nasal congestion for 20 years. More recently she had developed bronchitis, fatigue, nervousness, depression and peculiar eye symptoms. Study and testing by an allergist resulted in a diagnosis of "vasomotor rhinitis". Her symptoms became worse during the fall of 1982 and she received "3 rounds of antibiotics and 4 rounds of steroids".

---

†One study cited showed "absence of side effects when amphotericin B was given at a daily dose of 2 to 7 gm." In another study, "Patients received a total dose in excess of 1000 gm. without ill effects. *The lack of toxic effects observed with the tablets is in contrast with the marked toxicity, particularly at the renal level, which follows intravenous administration."*

I first saw Laura in January, 1983. I put her on my usual anti-candida program including diet, nystatin and nutritional supplements. She improved slightly. In March Laura developed an extensive rash. All medication was stopped including nystatin. The rash subsided. When she resumed the nystatin the rash returned. She stopped the nystatin and the rash again subsided.

Nizoral® was then prescribed and most of Laura's symptoms improved. Yet her nasal congestion continued. She also would develop a severe headache when she cheated on her diet.

Laura ran out of Nizoral® and in May, 1983, through a friend in France she obtained capsules of amphotericin B (Fungizone®). She took one-half of a 250 mg. capsule four times a day and sniffed tiny amounts of the powder.

Within two weeks she felt "much better". In a letter to me on August 3, 1983, Laura reported.

> "I'm doing great. I feel fantastically good, and my nose is clear for the first time in 20 years. I can even eat out in restaurants and cheat on my diet and not get into trouble.!"

I prescribe nystatin for nearly all of my patients with yeast-connected illness. Moreover, most of them improve on a comprehensive program which features nystatin, diet, lifestyle changes, supplemental nutrients and avoidance of chemical pollutants. In addition, some of my patients require immunotherapy (allergy vaccines or extracts). When a patient doesn't improve after several months on such a program (or even before) I often prescribe Nizoral® .

Yet because oral amphotericin B (without tetracycline) would provide an effective and safe alternative therapeutic weapon against Candida, I hope Squibb† will soon make it available for physicians and their patients in the United States. It seems to me that if oral amphotericin B helps the French and the Swiss it could do the same for Americans.

---

† On September 6, 1983, I received the following comments from Squibb about amphotericin B: "Until such time as there are well-controlled double-blinded multicenter studies of this use of amphotericin B, Squibb is unable to either endorse or encourage the oral use of this product. Additionally, we are very concerned to see that patients are sniffing the amphotericin B powder and must most vigorously discourage its use in this fashion and hope that you will do so also."

Physicians working to help patients with yeast-connected illness should be aware of

Other Candida species may cause problems: At the recent Birmingham Conference, Dr. Warren Pistey pointed out that *Candida albicans* is seen commonly in the everyday practice of pathology. Yet, at times it's hard to tell whether it is normal flora, an opportunist, or a pathogen. Dr. Pistey also noted that other species of candida, including *Candida tropicalis* and *Candida krusei,* are also found in some patients.

Charles M. Swaart (the man with a "still" in his intestines . . . see pages 229-230) recently wrote me and said, that it seems impossible for an M.D. to say or write the word 'Candida' without also using the word 'albicans.' He emphasized that *Candida albicans* isn't the only candida species that can cause problems. He referred especially to the book by H. I. Winner and R. Hurley, *Symposium on Candida Infections* (E. & S. Livingstone, Ltd., Edinburg and London).

New Methods of Studying and Treating Patients with Mold Sensitivity: In a paper presented at the annual seminar of the *Society for Clinical Ecology,* in November 1983, Sherry A. Rogers, M.D., told of her yeast and mold studies. I was fascinated by her presentation and feel her observations are relevant to any person interested in yeast-connected disorders.

In studies published in the July, 1982 and January, 1983 *Annals of Allergy,* Dr. Rogers showed that most laboratories, hospitals and allergists use the wrong culture media to identify common fungi in the air. She found that by making minor technical changes in the media, 32% more fungi were able to be identified (malt agar was substituted for the traditional Sabouraud's media)

---

these comments. However, as I have previously pointed out, the 1983 Physician's Desk Reference (page 1944) states that "oral administration of amphotericin B is usually well tolerated." (No adverse or toxic reactions are mentioned.)

Also, as previously noted, the studies of Montes, Cooper and associates found no evidence of toxicity from oral amphotericin B in contrast to the marked toxicity following intravenous administrations.

Candida albicans growing on mucous membranes leads to serious health disorders. Although oral nystatin and Nizoral® have proven effective in helping many individuals with these disorders, some individuals do not tolerate either drug.

Based on available evidence it seems to me that oral amphotericin B is a safe and effective anti-candida medication. Accordingly, I hope Squibb will encourage or support the "well-controlled double-blinded multicenter studies" of oral amphotericin B which they feel are needed.

"We used the results of studies to select antigens to test individually and showed before-and-after photos of diverse and severe recalcitrant conditions that were dramatically cleared with these newer fungal antigens. Discontinuing the injections was concomitant with recurrence of the conditions. An elimination diet was also required for most patients and likewise discontinuing the diet was concomitant with recurrence. The diet necessary for the majority was a *ferment-free diet*. That is, one free of products of fermentation such as yeast, bread, alcohol, cheese, vinegar, catsup, mayonnaise, mustard, salad dressing, chocolate and most factory foods."

Dr. Rogers also told of a study which has been accepted for publication in *The Annals of Allergy* in the spring of 1984. This study assessed the work-leisure-sleep, or 24-hour environment of patients for 13 months. Dr. Rogers said, in effect,

"The highlights of this study of 390 culture plates showed that the predominant class of fungi for every month was yeast. Yet, most previous studies fail to mention this because they only chart fungi which can be identified by genus and species name. Yeasts are not further differentiated by most mycologists because they require biochemical tests that take weeks to complete . . . *My studies show that we are barely scratching the surface when it comes to understanding the prevalence of yeasts in our environment.*"

In summarizing Dr. Rogers' presentation, it seems to me that the following points should be emphasized:

1. Immunotherapy with yeast and mold extract often helps, but it may not help as much as we would like.

2. *When it isn't effective, it may be because the mold antigens we use do not accurately represent the fungi which are bothering a particular patient.*

3. To more accurately obtain proper yeast and mold extracts for testing and treatment often requires cultures of the patient's home or workplace.

4. Instructions for obtaining such cultures can be obtained from:
   Mold Survey Service
   2800 West Genesee Street
   Syracuse, New York 13219

This laboratory will supply plates (Petri dishes with malt agar) and instructions for their exposure at $10 (U.S.) per plate.

Within four weeks after having mailed back the plates, your doctor will receive the results of the mycologist's findings including the type of mold that grew and the number of colonies present.

Selenium and other antioxidants: Information I've recently obtained from several sources suggests that a group of nutrients called *"antioxidants"* are important in restoring immune function and combatting what is termed "free radical pathology." Free radicals are sometimes "bad guys." Briefly, they appear to be promiscuously reactive molecules and molecular fragments which react aggressively with other molecules.

Although many free radical chemical reactions occur normally in the body and are necessary for health, other such reactions damage tissues. Substances which protect the body are called *free radical scavengers* or *antioxidants.* These include selenium, ascorbate (vitamin C), vitamin E, Beta carotene and glutathione.

The Food and Nutrition Board has recommended a dietary intake of 50 to 200 micrograms of selenium per day. However, some physicians feel a range of 100 to 300 micrograms may be optimal. Selenium-rich foods include butter, wheat germ, Brazil nuts, barley, scallops, lobster, shrimp and oats.

For further information on selenium, see the book *Trace Elements, Hair Analysis and Nutrition* by Richard A. Passwater, Ph.D., and Elmer M. Cranton, M.D., Keats Publishing Company, Inc., New Canaan, Ct., 1983; or the article "Biochemical-Pathology Initiated by Free Radicals, Oxidant Chemicals And Therapeutic Drugs In the Etiology of Chemical Hypersensitivity Disease," by Steven A. Levine, Ph.D. and Jeffrey H. Reinhardt. (Journal of Orthomolecular Psychiatry, Vol 12, #3, Pages 166-183, 1983)

Are selenium and other supplements important in strengthening the immune system and helping a person overcome yeast-connected illness? Although I can't answer this question with authority, a number of clinicians and researchers feel that such supplementation is appropriate and necessary, especially in patients who live in parts of the country where soil selenium is low.

Laboratory studies may help: The diagnosis and treatment of yeast-connected illness at this time (January, 1984) is based almost entirely on the typical history (see pages 17-33) followed by the response to an anti-candida program of treatment. Nevertheless, in some patients laboratory studies of various kinds may be helpful in corroborating the diagnosis of immune system disorders. Such studies may also help in structuring a more appropriate treatment program for patients with chronic health problems related to *Candida albicans*.

Immune system studies: Between May, 1981 and May, 1982, C. Orian Truss, M.D. and Max Cooper, M.D., of Birmingham, AL, carried out studies of T-lymphocytes including the ratio of helper cells to suppressor cells in patients with candida-related disorders. Abnormalities were found in many of these patients including some with chemical sensitivity (Truss, C. O., *Journal of Orthomolecular Psychiatry*, Volume 10, No. 4, page 235).

Alan Levin, M.D., San Francisco, told me recently that he had noted T-cell changes in patients with food and chemical sensitivity and "immune system dysregulation" induced by *Candida albicans*. Levin has especially noted changes in the helper/suppressor ratio. The usual ratio of helper cells to suppressor cells is 1.6 - 2.3 to 1. Patients with candida will often show a ratio below 1.3 to 1 or lower. Moreover, a ratio below 1.4 or 1.5 to 1 is suspicious of an immune system problem. In addition to changes in the ratio, the absolute number of T-cells is also often decreased in many patients with illness related to *Candida albicans*.

In January, 1984, I talked to Ed Winger, M.D., a pathologist (Immunodiagnostic Laboratory, 400 29th Street, Oakland, California 94609), about new laboratory tests that may help in studying patients with yeast-connected health problems. Dr. Winger commented,

> "The clinical diagnosis of yeast-related health disorders can sometimes be difficult. Serum tests for candida have been developed for patients with severe and life-threatening forms of candida. These patients have taught us that the testing techniques can help in making the proper diagnosis. New serum tests can indicate what type of antibodies the patient is making to fight candida.
>
> In patients with non-life threatening forms of candida, antibodies belonging to classes G and M (IgG and IgM) tend to be higher than the antibodies in non-infected persons while class A (IgA) tend to be lower.
>
> We can predict the likelihood that a patient has a candida-related health problem using these tests. They can be carried out at the time the diagnosis is suspected and then again after treatment is begun. Changes in antibody levels help confirm the diagnosis and help monitor the success of treatment."

Blood vitamin studies: Some individuals with yeast-connected illness (especially those with digestive problems) suffer from vitamin deficiencies. Such deficiencies are often related to a person's inability to absorb vitamins even though supplements are taken.

Blood studies may help in determining vitamin deficiencies or excesses. Such studies are reliably carried out in a number of laboratories including Vitamin Diagnostics, Incorporated (Dr. Herman Baker), Route 35 and Industrial Avenue, Cliffwood Beach, NJ 07735 and Monroe Medical Research Laboratory, Route 17, P.O. Box 1, Southfield, NY 10957, phone 914-351-5134 or 1-800-831-3133.

Mineral studies: To conquer candida and get well you need proteins, carbohydrates and fats. You also need vitamins and minerals. In determining your mineral status, examinations of your hair, blood and urine are sometimes appropriate.

Physicians interested in carrying out such studies can obtain further information from Doctors Data, 30 W. 101 Roosevelt Road, West Chicago, IL, phone: 1-800-323-2784 or 312-231-3649; MineraLab, Inc., P.O. Box 5012, Hayward, CA 94540, phone: 415-783-5622; Omega Tech Laboratory, Medical Director: Elmer Cranton, M.D., P.O. Box 1, Trout Dale, VA 24378, phone: 703-677-3103.

Amino acid studies: Amino acids combine in your body to form proteins. Recent clinical and laboratory studies suggest that some patients with chronic physical and mental illnesses including those who react to environmental chemicals show deficiencies or disturbances in their amino acids.

By collecting and analyzing 24 hour urine samples, data may be obtained that may serve as a guide to amino acid therapy (see *More on Amino Acids* pages 292-293).

Physicians interested in carrying out such studies can obtain further information from Bio Center Laboratory, 3715 East Douglas, Wichita, KS, phone: 1-800-835-3377; Bionostics, P.O. Drawer 400, Lisle, IL 60532 (Dr. John Pangborn, Ph.D., Director); Bio Science Laboratories, 150 Community Drive, P.O. Box 825, Great Neck, NY 11022, phone: 516-829-8000; Monroe Medical Research Laboratory, Route 17, P.O. Box 1, Southfield, NY 10975, phone: 914-351-5134 or 1-800-831-3133.

Fatty acid studies: Most Americans consume too much fat, especially fatty meats and hardened vegetables oils (found in margarines and most processed foods). But all fats aren't "bad guys" and some are important if your body is to function correctly. These fats are called "essential fatty acids" (see also page 141).

There are two series of essential fatty acids, the "omega 6" series starting with cis-linolenic acid and the "omega 3" series starting with alpha-linolenic acid. Both series can give rise to prostaglandins (PGs) which probably play key roles in brain function. According to studies carried out by Horrobin, cis-linolenic acid (found especially in evening primrose oil) along with large daily doses of vitamin B-6 (100-200 milligrams) seems to help patients with premenstrual syndrome (PMS.)

Although I haven't used such studies in my own practice I recently learned that "Essential Fatty Acid Profiles" can be determined by several laboratories including the Monroe Medical Research Laboratory, Route 17, P.O. Box 1, Southfield, NY 10975, phone 1-800-831-3133.

Yeast Toxins: When I gave a copy of the first edition of *The Yeast Connection* to one of my associates to review he commented,

> "I found your book interesting. Yet I'm wondering if there are studies which show that *Candida albicans* actually produces "toxins" that make people 'sick all over' "?

At the time I was unable to give him a satisfactory answer. But in late December, 1983, soon after the Birmingham symposium, *The Yeast-Human Interaction*, Phyllis Saifer, Editor of the Newsletter of the Society for Clinical Ecology commented,

> "As you know Dr. Kazuo Iwata of Tokyo presented a lot of material on yeast toxins at the Birmingham conference 2 weeks ago. But due to language difficulties I could catch only fragments of what he said. However I've just reviewed several of his scientific articles on yeast toxins. Here's a summary of his observations:
> Toxins from several candida strains
> 1. Suppress T & B cells both in number & function
> 2. Enhance vascular permeability
> 3. Promote the release of histamine
> 4. Induce anaphylactic reactions

Yeast-connected urticaria (hives): A famous allergist once announced at a national conference that he'd rather see a tiger come into his office than a patient with chronic urticaria. Yeasts aren't "the cause" of this devilishly difficult disorder, yet since my first candida patient in 1979 suffered from chronic urticaria and recovered completely (see page v), the subject interests me. Moreover, I successfully treated Robert (see pages 192-193) and 5 other patients with chronic hives using anticandida therapy.

The yeast-urticaria connection was clearly described by G. Holti in 1966 (*Symposium on Candida Infection*, ed. Winner H.L. and Hurley R., Edinburgh: Livingstone, 1966, p. 73-81) Holti studied 255 patients with chronic urticaria, and 49 of the group reacted to candida extract. Of these 49, 27 were "clinically cured" using oral and vaginal nystatin. An additional 18 overcame their urticaria when they followed a low yeast diet for several months. In 1970 James and Warrin (*British Journal of Dermatology*, 84,: 227, 1971) confirmed Holti's observations, and so did Alfred Zamm a Kingston, New York allergist and clinical ecologist in 1970 (see page 4).

More on Candida and Autism: (an anecdotal report) On January 7, 1984, I talked to Charles Swaart of Phoenix, AZ., who told me this fascinating story. (See pages 229 & 230 for a discussion of Mr. Swaart's experiences with candida)

> "Some months ago a woman called me to tell me about her 22 year old daughter who was diagnosed as having autism when she was a young child. For almost 20 years she required total care 24 hours a day. All the mother could do was feed her, keep her clean and shelter her. The child showed scant interest in outside surroundings and talked very little. At times she would act drunk and stagger and show other symptoms of intoxication.
>
> After reading the autism article by Don Campbell in the California paper (see page 197) she called my home and talked to my wife who told her more about candida. She went back to her doctor who ridiculed the idea. So she kept on talking and writing to my wife. Yet there was nothing my wife and I could do. Finally she called not long ago and told us her daughter was in the hospital with pneumonia and was receiving massive doses of antibiotics. She asked me if I would help her.
>
> So I wrote her doctor and sent him all sorts of materials about the relationship of *Candida albicans* to autism and other severe mental and nervous system symptoms. This finally convinced him and he put the young woman on Nizoral® in large doses. Since then she has shown a marked improvement in her mental status.

Incidentally, Mr. Swaart tells me he has just completed a manuscript of a book (tentatively titled *Endogenous Alcohol Syndrome*) on the relationship of candida to the "drunk disease" and is looking for a publisher.

More on PMS: *Does candida cause PMS?* No. Candida isn't THE cause of the premenstrual syndrome or other problems affecting women. *Yet, there's growing evidence (based on exciting clinical experiences of many physicians) that there is a yeast connection.* And by using measures to discourage candida colonization, many women with PMS improve . . . sometimes dramatically. Yet, obviously, as with many other disorders ranging from arthritis to depression, other therapies are needed, including nutritional therapy.

Here are recent references documenting the efficacy of nutritional therapy:

In an article in the July, 1983 *Journal of Reproductive Medicine*, Guy E. Abraham, M.D. reported that all types of PMS patients may benefit from extra magnesium and B complex vitamins. In addition, tension and anxiety improve with 200 to 800 mgs. of B-6 a day. Eating less refined sugar, dairy products and arachidonic acid (in animal fats) also appeared to be helpful.

Patients with bloating and weight gain were helped by extra B-6 and by reduced sugar, caffeine and salt intake. Those with breast tenderness obtained relief with large doses of vitamin E, while those with headache, dizziness and sugar craving were helped by essential fatty acids (from vegetable oils), magnesium, zinc and vitamins B-3, B-6 and C.

In another report (*Journal of the American College of Nutrition*, 2:115-122, 1983), Robert S. London, M. D. of Baltimore described controlled research studies using vitamin E. With vitamin E there was a significant improvement in the following symptoms: nervous tension, mood swings, irritability, anxiety, headache, craving for sweets, increased appetite, heart pounding, fatigue and dizziness or fainting, depression, forgetfulness, crying, confusion and insomnia. Doses ranging from 150 to 600 I.U. of vitamin E were used; 300/I.U. per day appeared to be optimal.

In still another report in the *Journal of Reproductive Medicine* (28:465-468, July, 1983), David F. Horrobin described five studies using evening primrose oil (EPO) in women with PMS. Daily doses varied from 4 to 8 capsules, each containing 0.5 grams of Efamol® brand EPO, which contains 9% gammalinolenic acid.

Significant improvement was observed in irritability, breast tenderness, ankle swelling, headache and depression. The author also suggested that addition of magnesium, zinc and vitamins B-3, B-6 and C resulted in an even greater response.

According to Leo Wollman, M.D., writing in the September, 1983 issue of *Cosmopolitan*, women need additional calcium especially during the 10 days prior to the onset of menstruation.

Marital Problems and Divorce: These unfortunate phenomena have been increasing in epidemic proportions during the past decade. Although the causes are multiple and complex, yeast-connected health disorders appear to play an important role.

Men with the "yeast problem" tend to be tired, irritable and depressed. They're often plagued by recurrent headaches and digestive disorders and their work productivity is reduced. Moreover, they may be troubled by prostatitis and a diminished sex drive.

Yeast-related disorders are especially devastating to women because yeast toxins affect hormone function. Recurrent or persistent vaginitis, menstrual irregularities, pain accompanying intercourse, fatigue, headaches, mood swings, depression and premenstrual tension occur commonly in the "yeast victim." Moreover, the problems of women are often aggravated by birth control pills, pregnancy and recurrent urinary tract infections.

Making a marriage work requires many things, including love, mutual respect and a lot of hard work. Even under ideal conditions, difficulties arise. So when one or both members of a union suffer from a yeast-connected health disorder, marital problems are an almost inevitable result.

Garlic May Help Control Yeasts†: Garlic has been widely used for medicinal purposes for centuries; for example, Virgil and Hippocrates mentioned it as a remedy for pneumonia and snake bite. In looking through the *Index Medicus*, I found numerous articles from the American and foreign literature describing the inhibitory action of garlic (Allium sativum) on candida organisms. Included

---

† Yeasts grow like bermuda grass. Plant parts include branches ("*mycelia*") and buds (*spores*). According to a candida researcher (who has taken garlic for his own yeast-connected health problems) garlic may harm as well as help. Although it kills yeast spores it may drive mycelial forms into the deeper tissues where they continue to release toxins and cause problems for their hosts.

among these was an article telling of the effect of garlic juice on two types of bacteria (*Staphyloccus areus and E.coli*) as well as on *Candida albicans*. "*Candida albicans* was found to be 'the most sensitive' of these three organisms to garlic juice.

Another paper commented,

> "Garlic possesses a broad antifungal activity, both on agar plates and in broth. Neither nystatin, nor amphotericin B . . . displayed such a high activity as garlic juice."

Still another article noted that all but 2 out of 26 strains of *Candida albicans* were sensitive to aqueous dilutions of garlic extract.

In spite of these studies . . . and there are many of them . . . Sanford Bolton and Gary Null and associates, writing in the *American Pharmacy (The Medical Uses of Garlic . . . Fact and Fiction,* August, 1982) pointed out that large scale controlled clinical trials of garlic still had never been conducted by the Food and Drug Administration. Moreover, such trials are time-consuming and extremely expensive. Accordingly, garlic, at the present time, might be considered as an orphan drug . . . a drug that has therapeutic application with little commercial potential.

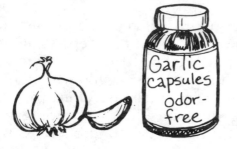

Garlic, like yogurt, seems to help eradicate candida spores in the intestinal tract. Moreover, several preparations of deodorized garlic possess anti-candida activity without retaining the offensive, garlic odor. Should you take garlic or garlic preparations to combat candida? I don't know and I hope further clinical studies and medical research will provide an answer.

More on Amino Acids: Amino acids are the "building blocks" found in proteins. There are 22 of them; some are essential while others are non-essential. According to John Pangborn, Ph.D.,† a specialist in the field, besides classical (acute) metabolism disorders, subclinical to subacute amino acid disorders are present in many diseases. Included among these are fatigue states, depres-

---

† Bionostics, Inc., P.O. Drawer 400, Lisle, IL 60532

sion, allergic-like reactions to foods, learning disabilities, neuroses, psychoses and seizure states.

My experience in studying and treating health disorders related to amino acid metabolic defects is extremely limited. Yet because some of the symptoms associated with amino acid disturbances are found in patients with yeast-connected health disorders (especially fatigue, depression and allergic-like reactions to foods) amino acid metabolism intrigues me.

This type of metabolism involves enzymes, mineral activators, co-enzymes (from vitamin precursors) and other factors. Rapid inexpensive chromatographic procedures are now being carried out by a number of laboratories to measure urine and plasma amino acids. Moreover, corrective supplements are now available including amino acids, keto acids, vitamins, minerals and digestive enzymes

Should your amino acid state be investigated? I don't know. Yet, if your health problems are yeast-connected and you have followed a comprehensive program of management for four months or longer and aren't improving, amino acid studies and appropriate therapy could help you.

Comments on Milk: During my twenties and early thirties I was bothered by recurrent abdominal pain and sinusitis. When I stopped drinking milk both health problems vanished. And during the last 25 years of my practice hundreds of my patients rid themselves of troublesome symptoms when they avoided milk.

Yet, in spite of my wariness of milk, I didn't usually restrict this beverage in my patients with yeast-connected health problems during the years 1979-1982. Then in the fall of 1983, after visiting with Shirley Lorenzani and Pat Connolly, I began to realize that the carbohydrate in milk (lactose) could promote yeast growth. Yet, in the first 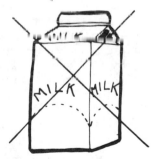 edition of *The Yeast Connection,* I included milk on both the *Candida Control Diet* and the *Low Carbohydrate Diet.*

Then on January 18, 1984, I received a letter from John A. Henderson, M.D. of San Diego who commented,

> "In this office we restrict milk because of the lactose content as well as the presence of molds. *Candida albicans* may not be able to ferment lactose but in individuals who break the lactose down into glucose and fructose, yeasts thrive on both of these sugars. There are approximately 12 grams of lactose in every eight ounces of milk and I hardly see the rationale for permitting candida patients to use milk in their diets."

Soon afterward, I telephoned John W. Rippon, Ph.D. and read him Dr. Henderson's comments. Dr. Rippon told me he agreed with Dr. Henderson. He also pointed out that intestinal bacteria and enzymes from the pancreas break down lactose and, in so doing, provide simple sugars for the candida to thrive on.

Based on these observations, *if your health problems are yeast-connected, avoid milk until your immune system improves and your candida is controlled.* Then you can cautiously experiment. (However, sugar-free yogurt preparations may be tolerated and may help lessen candida colonization in your digestive tract or vagina. See pages 266-267.)

Exercise: Everyone knows that exercise does all sorts of good things for you. And although I've talked briefly about exercise, I haven't emphasized its role in helping my patients strengthen their immune systems and conquer candida. So I feel the story of Maria will interest you.

On March 3, 1983, Maria wrote:

> "My awareness of allergy problems began in the fall of 1982 when we closed up our house for the winter. I began to develop severe headaches and depression that would come and go. I was confused and unable to sort out my thoughts. I developed paranoid feelings and thoughts of suicide kept popping into my head.
>
> "I reflected on my life and could find no psychological or familial reason for this. I was enjoying being at home and my husband, my children and I were relating well.
>
> "By what I consider an act of God, I found a neighbor who had experienced all sorts of allergies, including food and chemical sensitivities. She told me I was probably reacting to gas in my home. I had also noticed that my 2-year old had become very hyper and my infant was much crabbier than he had been up to that time. We experimented with turning off the gas and, amazingly, most of our symptoms disappeared.
>
> "Through experimentation, I've learned I feel better when I stay away from yeast-containing foods . . . less diarrhea and less fatigue. Yet, I continued to be bothered by diarrhea, stomach pains, nausea, irritability and an extreme craving for sweets and other foods as well. Please help."

Because of her chemical sensitivity, a history of vaginitis and a Candida Questionnaire score of 181, I put Maria on nystatin, a sugar-free, yeast-free diet and nutritional supplements. She improved steadily, although there were ups and downs in the ensuing months.

In January, 1984, Maria wrote:

> "I've gotten over the major hurdle in the treatment of my yeast problems. Since Christmas, I've felt more stable and healthier than I have in a long time. Moreover, I've been able to get off nystatin. I've also recently found I'm able to introduce offending foods into my diet, although I'm careful not to overdo it.
>
> *"I've also discovered that exercise play a major role in keeping me well . . . maybe the largest factor at this point.* I try to work out on weights, swim or exercise at least four times a week. As I begin to exercise, I can feel the tension and anger escape me and I feel more energy that day and the day after I work out."

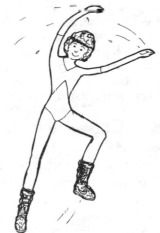

Maria's emphasis on the benefits she derived from exercise are impressive. Her story also illustrates the importance of other factors which played a role in strengthening her immune system and helping her get well. These included prayer, avoiding chemical pollutants, diet, nystatin, nutritional supplements, and avoiding sugar and yeast-containing foods.

More on Aspartame: Although aspartame is legal and is now being added to hundreds of foods and beverages, controversy surrounding its safety has been growing. For example in the January 13, 1984 issue of the Wall Street Journal Staff Reporter, Gary Putka said,

> "The Arizona Department of Public Health is testing soft drinks containing aspartame — for possible signs that the chemical may deteriorate into toxic levels of methyl alcohol under certain storage conditions."

Storing soft drinks containing aspartame in higher than normal temperatures was of special concern to these investigators. The possible adverse effects of aspartame were also recently discussed on several national television programs.

Yet, on February 10, 1984 I talked to Laura Jane Stevens of West Lafayette, Indiana, author of the forthcoming book, *A New Way to Sugar Free Cooking* (see page 314), who gave me a different point of view. Because sugar made her son, Jack, hyperactive for years, Laura worked to feed her family using sugar-free recipes. So when aspartame came along it helped her so much she read everything she could get her hands on (including many reports of F.D.A. research). Here are her comments:

> "The breakdown ingredients of aspartame which its detractors are talking about are commonly found in fruits and vegetables in even greater quantities.
>
> "Of course, aspartame may occasionally cause adverse effects, just as does any substance taken into the body, including commonly eaten foods. I'm aware of these food-induced reactions because I've experienced them; so have my children.
>
> "Nevertheless, I feel comfortable about using aspartame and recommending it to others. Naturally, aspartame, like anything we consume, (whether it's milk, bananas or peanuts!) should be taken in moderation. And if it disagrees or causes adverse reactions, it can be avoided."

So what do you do? You can make up your own mind. Here are my suggestions: (1) Avoid all refined sugar products until you've conquered your candida. Also avoid or limit fruits. (2) Even after you're well, sharply limit your intake of refined sugar. Although it tastes good, it isn't good for you. To sweeten foods where sugar is called for in the recipe, use fruits as suggested by Karen Barkie (see page 124). However, to repeat, *fruits should be avoided until your candida is under control. (3) Until you're well, when you must sweeten foods or beverages, use aspartame or saccharin . . . but don't go overboard.*

Mercury/Amalgam Toxicity: Several years ago, a friend of mine, J.W. Pyron, D.D.S., a preventive dentist of Cincinnati told me that silver/amalgam fillings contain significant amounts of mercury. As these fillings age, they apparently release mercury into the body. Since mercury is a toxic metal, according to Dr. Pyron it may produce symptoms in susceptible individuals.

Subsequently, I learned of the observations of Colorado dentist, Dr. Hal Huggins, and New York dentist, Dr. Jerome Mittelman, both of whom feel that mercury/amalgam fillings play a role in making a lot of people sick. More recently, I listened to an audio tape and heard comments by Roy Kupsinel, M.D., Michael F. Ziff, D.D.S. and James E. Hardy, D.M.D. These professionals feel that mercury/amalgam fillings cause chronic physical and mental disorders in some individuals. Interestingly enough, the "all over" symptoms they describe resemble those found in patients with yeast-connected health disorders.

To get other opinions on this subject, on January 27, 1984 I phoned Elmer Cranton, M.D., Phyllis Saifer, M.D. and Ken Gerdes, M.D. I asked each of them if they felt mercury/amalgam toxicity was contributing to the health problems of their patients with yeast-connected illness.

Their replies were similar. Each said in effect,

> "I've heard about this problem and the subject interests me. Yet, I haven't studied it sufficiently to provide you with an authoritative opinion as to its importance and significance."

I also called Dr. Pyron who commented,

> "I continue to be interested in mercury/amalgam toxicity. Yet how frequently it occurs and how important it is in causing health problems remains very controversial."

Because I'm open minded, even though I have made no attempt to evaluate my patients for mercury/amalgam toxicity, I felt I should bring up the subject. Moreover, I feel that individuals with severe yeast-connected health disorders, especially those who aren't improving, might well investigate the possibility that their mercury/amalgam fillings could be contributing to their health problems.

Those interested in learning more about mercury/amalgam toxicity can obtain further information by sending a stamped, self-addressed envelope to *The Toxic Element Research Foundation*, (Dr. Hal Huggins), P.O. Box 2589, Colorado Springs, CO 80906, *Kup's Comments*, published by Roy Kupsinel, M.D., P.O. Box 550, Oviedo, Florida 32765, or to the *Mittleman Newsletter*, 263 West End Avenue, #2-A, New York, New York 10023.

What Does "Orthomolecular" Mean: About 15 years ago Linus Pauling, Ph.D., a two-time winner of the Nobel Prize coined the term, "orthomolecular". And he published his now famous report entitled, "Orthomolecular Psychiatry" in *Science*, the journal of the American Association for the Advancement of Science. "Ortho" means to straighten. For example, the *ortho*donist straightens teeth, and the *ortho*pedist works to provide straight bones.

Pauling used the term *ortho*molecular to convey the idea that many chronic mental disorders could be corrected by "straightening" the concentration of molecules in the brain.

Dr. Pauling's approach represents a radical change from the usual medical and psychiatric approach which deals primarily with the use of synthetic drugs which aren't normally present in the body. Orthomolecular nutrition now is applied to every part of the body and recognizes that people are biochemically different and unique (as has been frequently emphasized by Roger J. Williams, Ph.D.).

Accordingly, in evaluating and treating patients with yeast-connected illness and other chronic health disorders, I try to "straighten" my patients. One of the ways I work to accomplish this goal is by helping them obtain the nutrients they need and avoid the toxic substances which contribute to their illnesses.

More on Nutrition: About ten years ago Dr. Jean Mayer of Boston pointed out that the average physician knows about as much about nutrition as his secretary — unless his secretary belongs to *Weight Watchers*. Then the physician is apt to know half as much! About the same time I saw an editorial in the *Southern Medical Journal* which pointed out that there had been a "blackout" in nutrition education in most medical schools.

Like my peers I spent more time during my residency treating disease than preventing it. And I knew nothing about many nutritional subjects that fascinate me today. Interestingly enough, much of what I've learned about nutrition through the years has come from non-medical publications.

These include *Executive Health*, an 8-page monthly commentary which discusses topics such as magnesium, vitamin C & backache, vitamin B-6, preventing alcoholism, exercise and many other topics you need to know about if you want to enjoy good health. Moreover, the editorial board of this publication includes two Nobel Prize winners plus other scientists and academicians with impeccable credentials.

Another authoritative source of nutrition information is the *Center for Science in the Public Interest*† (CSPI). This Washington, D.C. based organization (headed by Michael Jacobson, Ph.D.) deserves high marks. In my opinion *it ranks at the top of the list of organizations working to improve the quality of food offered to Americans.* I support this organization and during the past 10 years I've learned a lot from their publications including, especially, their illustrated, highly readable periodical *Nutrition Action.* (see also page 260).

Other excellent sources of nutrition information include the health food magazines, *Prevention, Best Ways, Let's Live* and *Your Good Health* which are now read by millions of subscribers. In *Prevention* I first read about the work of the late Henry Schroeder of Dartmouth College, the brilliant pioneer in the field of trace minerals. Through this same magazine I also learned of the work of Dr. Tom Brewer. This crusading obstetrician had worked untiringly to stress the importance of feeding mothers a good diet during pregnancy rather than limiting their weight and treating them with "water pills". Also, through articles in the health food magazines, I first learned that my adult patients, (especially females,) needed calcium and magnesium supplements to prevent their bones from disintegrating. Moreover this was 7 or 8 years before I read an editorial in the *New England Journal of Medicine* making similar recommendations.

But health food magazines aren't the only sources of nutrition information. Increasingly, informative articles are appearing in other widely read periodicals including *Reader's Digest, Woman's Day, Cosmopolitan, New Woman, Family Circle, Ladies Home Journal, the Rotarian* and many others. Such articles usually emphasize that better health doesn't always come from more doctoring, more drugs and more hospitals. Instead it is achieved from better nutrition, exercise, stopping smoking and changing your lifestyle.

If you suffer from yeast-connected health problems keep reading, studying and learning about nutrition and about yourself and your response and reactions to different foods. As I've noted previously (pages 67-72) *you are unique and your dietary requirements, tolerances and sensitivities differ considerably from those of other people (including members of your own family.)*

As much as I've worked to standardize my dietary instructions

I've found that *no rules can be laid down which suit every patient*. Nevertheless, I feel you'd like to know what I tell my patients today (February 10, 1984):

1. Make sure your diet is nutritionally adequate with fresh foods from a wide variety of sources.
2. *Diversify or rotate your foods.* (See pages 129-130). Food intolerances, sensitivities or allergies develop more commonly in those who eat the same foods every day. Also, by rotating your diet you'll be better able to identify foods that disagree with you.
3. *Avoid all refined carbohydrates,* including sugar, corn syrup, dextrose and fructose. Also avoid honey, maple syrup and date sugar. Feeding sugar and simple carbohydrates to candida organisms is like pouring kerosene on a fire.
4. *Avoid refined, processed and fabricated foods.* Such foods usually contain sugar, yeasts and other hidden ingredients that may bother you. Moreover, other important nutrients including essential fatty acids, vitamins and minerals have been removed from many of these foods. In addition harmful (or potentially harmful) ingredients have been substituted — as for example, hardened vegetable oils and additives of various types.
5. During the early weeks of your diet *avoid fruits and milk* as the carbohydrates in these foods seem to encourage candida growth.
6. Since whole fruits are good food, as you improve try rotating them back into your diet and see if you tolerate them.
7. During the early weeks of your diet *avoid all yeast and mold containing foods.* As you improve you may find you can eat some of these foods (see also page 94).
8. Eat sugar-free *yogurt* (see pages 251, 266-267) and take nutritional supplements including vitamins, minerals and essential fatty acids.
9. If you don't improve on the dietary program outlined above, *temporary restriction of all carbohydrates* may be tried (see the *Low Carbohydrate Diet*). Yet, since complex carbohydrates provide so many essential nutrients, I do not permanently limit them.

40

Postscript

Since I first learned of the relationship of candida albicans to human illness, my life and my practice have changed dramatically. I can hardly wait to get to my office each day because I know I'll be seeing people I can help. Many of them complain of so many symptoms they've been labeled "hypochondriacs" Others with supposedly incurable diseases have been told "You'll have to learn to live with this condition." Yet, in the last four years, I've been able to help hundreds of long-suffering adult patients. Moreover, my experiences are being duplicated by many other physicians.

Although yeast-connected illness rarely causes sudden death, it leads to suffering, disability and disease which can last for decades. And it often shortens the life of its victims.

More recently I've become excited over the relationship of candida to health problems in children, especially (1) recurrent ear problems, (2) hyperactivity and behavior problems in preschool and early schoolage children, (3) problems in teenagers, including underachievement in school, depression, hostility, anti-social behavior, alcoholism, use of narcotics, traffic accidents and suicide.

As I've repeatedly pointed out, candida isn't "the cause" of those problems; yet my observations in treating a limited number of such youngsters make me feel that all of these problems are yeast-connected.

One reviewer of *The Yeast Connection* commented,

> "I like your book, but I can't help wishing that it was a more scientific endeavor and more medical research was available to give positive proof of the relationship of candida to human illness."

I can understand such a point of view, and I realize that nystatin and a special diet won't cure every human ailment. Yet, along with hundreds of American physicians and thousands of patients, I've found that an anti-candida program helps many frustrated, discouraged, sick people regain their health.

I freely acknowledge that many questions remain unanswered and I hope scientists and researchers will tackle them in the months and years to come. But, to repeat, *I'm excited.* And whether you're a physician, yeast victim or interested bystander, I hope *The Yeast Connection* will interest and help you, and you'll share in my excitement and join me in "spreading the word."

More Research Needed

I also hope you'll join me in supporting research which may help you and others with illness related to *Candida albicans.* Growing numbers of grateful patients who have benefitted from the pioneer work of Dr. C. Orian Truss have started an IRS approved public foundation to provide funds for research into the underlying causes and effects of this problem (yeast-connected illness).

Today, a laboratory has been built behind Dr. Truss' offices so he can direct ongoing research. In addition, several projects have been funded with internationally recognized scientists at the Medical College at the University of Alabama in Birmingham.

At the December, 1983 symposium on Human-Yeast Interaction in Birmingham, Dr. Sidney Baker pointed out that much of the research on *Candida albicans* has been carried out in the past in laboratories studying the basic biology of fungi. Yet, little attention has been paid to unraveling some of the clinical aspects of this problem. *Today, Dr. Truss' laboratory is really the only one whose focus is in that direction.* It is a tiny operation especially when it's compared to medical research funded by the drug companies..

Dr. Baker urged physicians, grateful patients—anyone and everyone—to contribute to the Critical Illness Research Foundation, 2614 Highland Avenue, Birmingham, Alabama 35205, and he commented,

> "It would speed the work of this genius and be good for everybody in return—and provide answers for some of our still unanswered questions."

I agree and I've just sent a contribution to this foundation and hope you'll do the same.

41

References

1. Crook, W.G.: "The Coming Revolution in Medicine." Journal of the Tennessee Medical Association, 76:145-149, 1983.
2. Rippon, J.W.: MEDICAL MYCOLOGY (2nd Edition). Philadelphia, W.B. Saunders, 1982.
3. Odds, F.C.: CANDIDA AND CANDIDOSIS. Baltimore, University Park Press, 1979.
4. Lucas, P.L., Macdonald, F., Peters, D.W. and Plumlee, L.A.: "Serological Identification of an Unrecognized Form of Candidosis with Acquired Immunodeficiency." Submitted for publication, 1983.
5.a. Crook, W.G.: CAN YOUR CHILD READ? IS HE HYPERACTIVE? Jackson, Tennessee, Professional Books, 1977 (revised edition), pps.150-155.
   b. Crook, W.G.: "Can What a Child Eats Make Him Dull, Stupid or Hyperactive?" Journal of Learning Disabilities, 13:53-58, 1980.
   c. Crook, W.G.: "Diet and Hyperactivity." Clinical Pediatrics (Letters), 68:300, 1981.
6. Cheraskin, E., Ringsdorf, W.M., Jr., Ramsay, R.R., Jr.: "Sucrose, Neutrophilic Phagocytosis and Resistance to Disease." Dental Survey, 52:46-48, 1976.
7. Prinz, R.J., Roberts, W.A., Hantman, E.: "Dietary Correlates of Hyperactive Behavior in Children." J. Consult. Clin. Psychol., 48:769, 1980.
8-a. Schoenthaler, S.: "The Effect of Sugar on the Treatment and Control of Anti-Social Behavior: A Double-Blind Study of an Incarcerated Juvenile Population." The International Journal for Biosocial Research, 3:1, 1982.
   b. Guenther, R.M.: "The Role of Nutritional Therapy in

Alcoholism Treatment." The International Journal for Biosocial Research, 4:5, 1983.

c. Warden, N., Duncan, M., Sommars, E.: "Nutritional Changes Heighten Children's Achievement: A 5-Year Study." The International Journal for Biosocial Research, 3:72, 1982.

9. PHYSICIANS DESK REFERENCE. Oradell, N.J., Medical Economics Co., 1983, p.1942.

10. Mandell, M.: DR. MANDELL'S 5-DAY ALLERGY RELIEF SYSTEM. New York, Pocket Books, 1979.

11. Cheraskin, E., Ringsdorf, W.M., Jr.: "How Much Refined Carbohydrate Should We Eat?" Amer. Lab., 6:31-35, 1974.

12. Brody, J.: JANE BRODY'S NUTRITION BOOK. New York, W.W. Norton & Co., 1981.

13. Crook, W.G.: TRACKING DOWN HIDDEN FOOD ALLERGY. Jackson, Tennessee, Professional Books, 1980.

14. Sterrett, F.S.: "How Safe is Long Island Drinking Water?" LONG ISLAND PEDIATRICIAN, Summer 1982 (published by Nassau County Medical Center, 2201 Hempstead Turnpike, East Meadow, New York.)

15. Hippocrates. As quoted by Bell, I.R.: CLINICAL ECOLOGY. Bolinas, Calif., Common Knowledge Press, 1982, p.7.

16. Schroeder, H.: TRACE ELEMENTS AND MAN. Old Greenwich, Connecticut, Devon-Adair, 1973.

17. Higgs, J.M., Wells, R.S.: "Chronic Muco-Cutaneous Candidiasis: New Approaches to Treatment." British Journal of Dermatology, 89:179, 1973.

18-a. Whedon, G.D.: "Osteoporosis." (Ed) The New England Journal of Medicine, 305:397-399, 1981.

b. Spencer, H.: "Osteoporosis: Goals of Therapy." Hospital Practice, March, 1982, pp.131-151.

c. Ulene, A.: "The Great Bone Robbery-Calcium: The Woman's Mineral." Family Circle, September, 1981, pp 67-68, 120.

19. Cheraskin, E., Ringsdorf, W.M., Jr., Ramsay, R.R., Jr.: "Sucrose, Neutrophilic Phagocytosis and Resistance to Disease." Dental Survey, 52:46-48, 1976.

20-a. Horrobin, D.F.: "Alcohol—Blessing and Curse of Mankind!" Executive Health, Vol. XVII, #9, June, 1981.

b. Horrobin, D.F.: PROSTAGLANDINS: PHYSIOLOGY, PHARMACOLOGY AND CLINICAL SIGNIFICANCE. Montreal, Eden Press, 1978.

c. Rudin, D.O.: "The Dominant Diseases of Modernized Societies as Omega-3 Essential Fatty Acid Deficiency Syndrome: Substrate Beriberi." MEDICAL HYPOTHESES, 8:241-242, 1982.

d. Rudin, D.O.: As quoted by Steven, L.J.: THE COMPLETE BOOK OF ALLERGY CONTROL. ("Looking at Your Essential Fatty Acids") New York, Macmillan, 1983.

21. Pauling, L.: "On Vitamin C and Infectious Diseases." Executive Health, Vol. 19, #4, 1983.

22. Cheraskin, E.: "The Name of the Game is the Name." In Williams, R.J. and Kalita, B.K.: A PHYSICIANS HANDBOOK ON ORTHOMOLECULAR MEDICINE, New York, Pergamon Press, 1977, pp. 40-44.

23. Cheraskin, E. and Ringsdorf, W.M., Jr.: PREDICTIVE MEDICINE. New Canaan, Connecticut, Keats Publishing, Inc., 1973.

24. Rea, W.: "Cardiovascular Disease Triggered by Foods and Chemicals." In Gerrard, J.W. (ed): FOOD ALLERGY: NEW PERSPECTIVES. Springfield, Illinois, Charles C. Thomas, 1980, pp. 99-143.

25-a. Levin, A.S., McGovern, J.J., LeCam, L.L., et al: "Immune Complex Mediated Vascular Inflammation in Patients With Food and Chemical Allergies." Annals of Allergy, 47:138, 1981.

b. McGovern, J.J., Lazaroni, J.A., Hicks, M.F., et al: "Food and Chemical Sensitivity. Clinical and Immunological Correlates." Arch. Otolaryngology (in press).

26. Williams, R.: PHYSICIANS HANDBOOK OF NUTRITIONAL SCIENCE, Springfield, Illinois, Charles C. Thomas, 1975, Chapter 9.

27-a. Baker, S.M.: UPDATE, Vol. 1, #1, July, 1980. (A quarterly Digest of Information and Ideas on the Psychological and Biological Basis of Human Behavior and Development, published by The Gesell Institute of Human Development, 310 Prospect St., New Haven, Connecticut 06511.)

b. Baker, S.M.: UPDATE, Vol. 2 #5, December, 1982.

28. Schroeder, H.: "Pure Food is Poor Food." Prevention, July, 1975, pps.124-136.

29. Cameron, E., Pauling, L.: CANCER AND VITAMIN C. New York, New York, W.W. Norton and Co., 1979, pp.108-111.

30. Anah, C., Jarike, L., Baig, H.: "High Dose Ascorbic Acid in Nigerian Asthmatics." Journal of Allergy and Clinical Immunology (Allergy Abstract Section), 62:5, 1981.

31. Cousins, N.: ANATOMY OF AN ILLNESS. New York, New York, W.W. Norton and Co., 1979.

32. Randolph, T.G., Moss, R.W.: AN ALTERNATIVE APPROACH TO ALLERGIES. New York, Lippincott & Crowell, 1980, p. 185.

33. Worthen, D.B.: Personal communication, March 29, 1983. (Chief of Information Services, Norwich Eaton Pharmaceuticals, Inc., Norwich, New York.)

34-a. Rowe, A.H., Sr.: "Allergic Toxemia and Migraine Due to Food Allergy." California West. Med., 33, 785, 1930.

b. Randolph, T.G.: "Allergy as a Causative Factor of Fatigue, Irritability and Behavior Problems in Children." J. of Pediatrics, 31:560, 1947.

c. Crook, W.G., Harrison, W.W., Crawford, S.E., Emerson, B.S.: "Systemic Manifestations Due to Allergy. Report of Fifty Patients and a Review of the Literature on the Subject (Allergic Toxemia and the Allergic Tension-Fatigue Syndrome)." Pediatrics, 27:790, 1961.

d. Gerrard, J.W., Heiner, D.C., Ives, E.J., Hardy, L.W.: "Milk Allergy: Recognition, Natural History, and Management." Clinical Pediatrics, 2:634, 1963.

e. Deamer, W.C.: "Pediatric Allergy: Some Impressions Gained Over a 37-year Period." Pediatrics, 48:930, 1971.

f. Crook, W.G.: "Food Allergy . . . The Great Masquerader." Pediatric Clinics of North America, 22: 227-238, 1975.

g. Rapp, D.J., Fahey, D.J.: "Allergy and Chronic Secretory Otitis Media." Pediatric Clinics of North America, 22: 259-264, 1975.

h. McGovern, J.P., Haywood, T.J., Fernandez, A.A.: "Allergy and Serous Otitis Media." Journal of American Medical Association, 200:124, 1967.

i. Deamer, W.C., Gerrard, J.W., Speer, F.: "Cow's Milk Allergy: A Critical Review." The Journal of Family Practice, 9:223-232, 1979.

35. Ogle, K., Bullock, J.D.: "Children with Allergic Rhinitis and/or Bronchial Asthma Treated with Elimination Diet: A

Five-Year Follow-up." Annals of Allergy, 44:273, 1980.

36. Speer, F.: ALLERGY OF THE NERVOUS SYSTEM. Springfield, Illinois, Charles C. Thomas, 1970.

37-a. Clein, N.W.: "Cow's Milk Allergy in Infants." Pediatric Clinics of North America, 1:949, 1954.

b. Matsumura, T., et. al.: "Significance of Food Allergy in the Etiology of Orthostatic Albuminuria." Journal of Asthma Research, 3:325, 1966.

38. McGee, C.T.: "How to Survive Modern Technology." Alamo, California, Ecology Press, 1979, p.11.

39. Crook, W.G.: "Adolescent Behavior." Clinical Pediatrics (Letters), 21:501, 1982.

40. Landers, A.: "Parents Should Give Help and Advice About Sex." Memphis Commerical Appeal, Section B., page 10, September 28, 1981.

41. Rosenberg, E.W., Belew, P.W., Skinner, R.B., Jr., Crutcher, N.: (Letters) The New England Journal of Medicine, 308:101, 1983.

42. Miller, J.B.: "Relief of Premenstrual Symptoms, Dysmenorrhea, and Contraceptive Tablet Intolerance." The Journal of the Medical Association of the State of Alabama, 44:14, 1974.

43. Mabray, C.R., Burditt, M.L., Martin, T.C., Jaynes, C.R., Hayes, J.R.: "Treatment of Common Gynecologic Endocrinologic Symptoms by Allergy Management Procedures." Obstetrics & Gynecology, Vol. 59, No. 5, 1982.

44. Kirkpatrick, C.H., Sohnle, P.G.: "Chronic Mucocutaneous Candidiasis." From IMMUNODERMATOLOGY, edited by Digun Eafai and Robert A. Good. Plenum Publishing Corporation, 1981, p. 495.

45. Hofstra, W., de Vries-Hospers, H.G., van der Waaij, D.: "Concentrations of Nystatin in Faeces after Oral Administration of Various Doses of Nystatin." Infection, 7:166-169, 179.

46-a. Miller, J.B.: "The Management of Food Allergy." In Gerrard, J.W. (ed.): FOOD ALLERGY: NEW PERSPECTIVES. Springfield, Ill., Charles C. Thomas, 1980, pp.274-282.

b. Sandberg, D.H.: "Renal Disease Related to Hypersensitivity to Foods." In Gerrard, J.W.: FOOD ALLERGY: NEW PERSPECTIVES, pp. 157-164.

   c. Rapp, D.J.: "Hyperactivity and the Tension-Fatigue Syndrome." In Gerrard, J. W.: FOOD ALLERGY: NEW PERSPECTIVES, PP.201-204.

   d. Hilsen, J.M.: "Dietary Control of the Hyperactive Child." The Long Island Pediatrician, Summer, 1982, pp. 25-32.

   e. O'Shea, J., Porter, S.F.: "Double-Blind Study of Children with Hyperkinetic Syndrome Treated with Multi-Allergen Extract Sublingually." Journal of Learning Disabilities, Vol. 14, #4, April, 1981.

47. Rinkel, H.J., Lee, C.H., Brown, D.W., Willoughby, J.W., Williams, J.M.: "The Diagnosis of Food Allergy." Arch. of Otolaryngology, 79:71, 1964.

48-a. Krueger, A.P.: "Air Ions as Biological Agents—Fact or Fancy?" (Part I) Immunology & Allergy Practice, Vol. 4, #4, pp. 129-140, 1982.

   b. Krueger, A.P.: "Air Ions as Biological Agents—Fact or Fancy? (Part II)". Immunology & Allergy Practice, Vol. 4 #5, pp. 173-183, 1982.

49. Soyka, F.: THE ION EFFECT. New York, E.P. Dutton & Co., Inc., 1977.

50. Davis, D.R.: "Using Vitamin A Safely." Osteopathic Medicine, 3:31-43, 1978.

51-a. Truss, C.O.: "Tissue Injury Induced by Candida Albicans: Mental and Neurologic Manifestations." The Journal of Orthomolecular Psychiatry, 7:17-37, 1978.

   b. Truss, C.O.: "Restoration of Immunologic Competence to Candida Albicans." The Journal of Orthomolecular Psychiatry, 9:287-301, 1980.

   c. Truss, C.O.: "The Role of Candida Albicans in Human Illness." The Journal of Orthomolecular Psychiatry, 10:228-238, 1981.

52. Truss, C.O.: THE MISSING DIAGNOSIS. P.O. Box 26508, Birmingham, Ala. 35226, 1983.

53. Crook, W.G.: (Letters) J. of Orthomolecular Psychiatry, 12:34-36, 1983.

54. Cathcart, R.F., III: "Vitamin C Function in AIDS". Medical Tribune, July 13, 1983.

55. Kirkpatrick, C.H., Alling, D.W.: "Treatment of Chronic Oral Candidiasis with Clotrimazole Troches." The New England Journal of Medicine, 299: 1201-1203, 1978.

42

Reading list

(*Denotes books of special interest to Physicians)

Allergy, Immunology, Clinical Ecology and Environmental Medicine

Bell, I.R.: CLINICAL ECOLOGY (A New Medical Approach to Environmental Illness). Bolinas, California, Common Knowledge Press, 1982.*

*Dickey, L.: CLINICAL ECOLOGY. Springfield, Illinois, Charles C. Thomas, 1975.

Faelten, S. and Editors of *Prevention* Magazine: ALLERGY SELF-HELP BOOK. Emmaus, Pennsylvania, Rodale Press.

Forman, R.: HOW TO CONTROL YOUR ALLERGIES. New York, Larchmont Books, 1979.

Frazier, C.A.: COPING WITH FOOD ALLERGY. New York, The New York Times Book Co., 1974.

Gerrard, J.W. (Ed): FOOD ALLERGY: NEW PERSPECTIVES. Springfield, Illinois, Charles C. Thomas, 1980.

Glasser, R.T.: THE BODY IS THE HERO. New York, Random House, 1976.

Golos, N., Golbitz, F.: COPING WITH YOUR ALLERGIES. New York, Simon and Schuster, 1978.

Golos, N., Golbitz, F.: IF THIS IS TUESDAY IT MUST BE CHICKEN, 1981. Available from: Human Ecology Research Foundation of the Southwest, 12110 Webbs Chapel Road, Suite 305 E., Dallas, Texas 75234.

*Hare, F.: THE FOOD FACTOR IN DISEASE. London, Longmans, Green and Co., Vols. 1 & 2, 1905.

Ilg, F.L., Ames, L.B., Baker, S.M.: CHILD BEHAVIOR. New York, Harper & Row, 1981.

Jones, M.: THE ALLERGY COOKBOOK, Emmaus, Pennsylvania, Rodale Press, 1984.

Levin, A., Dadd, D.L.: CONSUMER GUIDE FOR THE CHEMICALLY SENSITIVE. 1982. (Available from: Alan S. Levin, 450 Sutter, Suite 1138, San Francisco, Ca. 84105).

Levin, A. S. and Zellerbach, M.: TYPE 1/TYPE 2 ALLERGY RELEASE PROGRAM. Jeremy D. Tarcher, Inc., Los Angeles. Distributed Houghton Mifflin Company, Boston, Massachussetts, 1983.

Mackarness, R.: EATING DANGEROUSLY. New York, Harcourt Brace & Jovanovich, 1976.

Mackarness, R.: CHEMICAL VICTIMS. London, Pan Books, 1980.

Mackarness, R.: LIVING SAFELY IN A POLLUTED WORLD. New York, Stein & Day, 1981.

Mandell, M., Scanlon L.: DR. MANDELL'S 5-DAY ALLERGY RELIEF SYSTEM. New York, Pocket Books, 1979.

Mandell, M.: DR. MANDELL'S LIFETIME ARTHRITIS RELIEF SYSTEM. New York, Coward-McCann, 1983.

*Miller, J.: FOOD ALLERGY (Provocative Testing and Injection Therapy). Springfield, Illinois, Charles C. Thomas, 1972.

Nichols, V.: COOKBOOK AND EATING GUIDE. Xenia, Ohio 45385, 3350 Fair Oaks Drive.

*Philpott, W.H. and Kalita, B.K.: BRAIN ALLERGIES. New Canaan, Connecticut, Keats Publishing, Inc., 1980.

Randolph, T.G.: HUMAN ECOLOGY AND SUSCEPTIBILITY TO THE CHEMICAL ENVIRONMENT. Springfield, Ill., Charles C. Thomas, 1962.

Rapp, D.J.: ALLERGIES AND THE HYPERACTIVE CHILD. New York, Cornerstone, 1980.

Rapp, D.J.: ALLERGIES AND YOUR FAMILY. New York, Sterling, 1981.

Rippere, V.: THE ALLERGY PROBLEM: Why People Suffer and What Should Be Done. Thorson Publishers, Ltd., Wellingborough Northamptonshire, England, 1983.

Small, B.: THE SUSCEPTIBILITY REPORT. Deco-Plans, Inc. P. O. Box 870, Plattsburgh, New York, 12901 (in Canada, P. O. Box 3000, Cornwall, Ontario K6H 5R8).

Rockwell, S.: COPING WITH CANDIDA (A handbook of recipes). P. O. Box 15181, Seattle, Washington.

Small, B.&B.: SUNNYHILL. Goodwood, Ontario, Canada, Small & Associates, 1980.

Smith, L.H.: IMPROVING YOUR CHILD'S BEHAVIOR CHEM-

ISTRY. Englewood Cliffs, New Jersey, Prentice-Hall, 1976.

*Speer, F.: ALLERGY OF THE NERVOUS SYSTEM. Springfield, Ill., Charles C. Thomas, 1970.

*Speer, F.: FOOD ALLERGY. Littleton, Mass., PSG Publishing Co., Inc. 1983 (2nd edition).

Soyka, F., with Edmonds, A.: THE ION EFFECT. New York, Bantam Books, 1980.

Stevens, L.J. and G.E., Stoner, R.B.: HOW TO FEED YOUR HYPERACTIVE CHILD. New York, Doubleday, 1977.

Stevens, L.J., Stoner, R.B.: HOW TO IMPROVE YOUR CHILD'S BEHAVIOR THROUGH DIET. New York, Doubleday, 1979.

Stevens, L.J.: THE COMPLETE BOOK OF ALLERGY CONTROL. New York, MacMillan Publishing Co., 1983.

Truss, C.O.: THE MISSING DIAGNOSIS. 1983. (Available from P.O. Box 26508, Birmingham, Ala. 35226.)

Yoder, E.R.: A GUIDE FOR AN ALLERGEN-FREE ELIMINATION DIET, 1982. (Available from: Healthful Living Publishers, P.O. Box 563, Goshen, Ind., 44526.)

Wunderlich, R. and Kalita, D.: CANDIDA ALBICANS AND THE HUMAN CONDITION. New Canaan, Connecticut, Keats Publishing, Inc., 1984.

Wunderlich, R. and Kalita, D.: NOURISHING YOUR CHILD. New Canaan, Connecticut, Keats Publishing, Inc. 1984.

Zamm, A.V. with Gannon, R.: WHY YOUR HOUSE MAY ENDANGER YOUR HEALTH. New York, Simon and Schuster, 1980.

Nutrition and Preventive Medicine

Abrahamson, E.M., Pezet, A.W.: BODY, MIND, AND SUGAR. New York, Avon, 1951.

Banick, A. E. (with Carlson Wade): YOUR WATER AND YOUR HEALTH. New Canaan, Connecticut, Keats Publishing, Inc. 1981.

Bland, J.: NUTRAEROBICS: The Complete Individualized Nutrition and Fitness Program for Life After Thirty. San Francisco, Harper & Row, 1983.

Bland, J.: YOUR HEALTH UNDER SIEGE: Using Nutrition to Fight Back. Brattleboro, Vermont, Stephen Green, 1981.

Brewster, L., Jacobson, M.F.: THE CHANGING AMERICAN DIET, 1978. Available from CSPI Publications, 1755 S Street, N.W., Washington, D.C. 20009.

311

Brody, J.: JANE BRODY'S NUTRITION BOOK. New York, W.W. Norton and Co., 1981.

Brody, J.: THE NEW YORK TIMES GUIDE TO PERSONAL HEALTH. New York, Harper & Row, 1982.

Burros, M.F.: KEEP IT SIMPLE: 30-MINUTE MEALS FROM SCRATCH. New York, William Morrow & Co., Inc., 1981.

Cameron, E., Pauling, L.: CANCER AND VITAMIN C. New York, W.W. Norton & CO., 1979.

Cheraskin, E., Ringsdorf, W.M., Jr. and Brescher, A.: PSYCHO-DIETETICS. New York, Bantam Books, 1974.

Cheraskin, E., Ringsdorf, W.M., Jr., Sisley, E.L.: THE VITAMIN C CONNECTION. New York, Harper & Row, 1983.

Cleave, T.L.: THE SACCHARINE DISEASE. New Canaan, Connecticut, Keats Publishing, Inc., 1975.

Cousins, N.: ANATOMY OF AN ILLNESS. New York, Bantam Books, 1981.

Dufty, W.: SUGAR BLUES. Nutri-Books Corp., P.O. Box 358, Denver, Col. 80217.

Durk, P., Shaw, S.: LIFE EXTENSION. New York, Warner Books. 1982.

EXECUTIVE HEALTH (a monthly newsletter). (Pickfair Bldg., Rancho Santa Fe., Ca. 92067.

Fredericks, C.: PROGRAM FOR LIVING LONGER. New York, Simon & Schuster, 1983.

Fredericks, C.: PSYCHO-NUTRITION. New York, Grosset & Dunlap, 1976.

Goldbeck, N. and D.: THE SUPERMARKET HANDBOOK: ACCESS TO WHOLE FOODS. New York, Harper & Row, 1973.

Goodwin, M., Pollen, G.: CREATIVE FOOD EXPERIENCES FOR CHILDREN, 1980. CSPI Publications, 1755 S Street, N.W., Washington, D.C. 20009.

Guenther, R.: A NUTRITIONAL GUIDE TO THE PROBLEM DRINKER. New Canaan, Connecticut, Keats Publishing, Inc.

Hall, R.H.: FOOD FOR NOUGHT. New York, Harper & Row, 1977.

Hausman, P.: JACK SPRAT'S LEGACY: THE SCIENCE AND POLITICS OF FAT AND CHOLESTEROL. (Richard Marek, 1981). Available from CSPI Publications, 1755 S Street, N.W., Washington, D.C. 20009.

Hoffer, A., Walker, M.: ORTHOMOLECULAR NUTRITION. New

Canaan, CT., Keats Publishing Co., 1978.

Hunter, B.T.: FACT/BOOK ON FOOD ADDITIVES AND YOUR HEALTH. New Canaan, Connecticut, Keats Publishing, Inc., 1972.

Hunter, B.T.: THE GREAT NUTRITION ROBBERY. New York, Charles Scribner's Sons, 1978.

Hunter, B.T.: THE SUGAR TRAP & HOW TO AVOID IT. Boston, Houghton Mifflin Co., 1982.

Jacobson, M.F.: EATER'S DIGEST: THE CONSUMER'S FACT BOOK OF FOOD ADDITIVES. (New York, Doubleday Anchor Books, 1976.) Available from CSPI Publications, 1755 S Street, N.W., Washington, D.C. 20009.

Jones, S.: CRYING BABY, SLEEPLESS NIGHTS. New York, Warner Books, 1983.

Katz, D., Goodwin, M.: FOOD: WHERE NUTRITION, POLITICS AND CULTURES MEET, 1976. CSPI Publications, 1755 S Street, N.W., Washington, D.C. 20009.

Keough, C.: WATER FIT TO DRINK. Emmaus, Pa., Rodale Press, 1980.

Kinsella, S.: FOOD ON CAMPUS, A RECIPE FOR ACTION (Emmaus, Pa., Rodale Press, 1978). Available from CSPI Publications, 1755 S Street, N.W., Washington, D.C. 20009.

Lansky, V.: THE TAMING OF THE C.A.N.D.Y. MONSTER. Wayzata, MN., Meadowbrook Press, 1978.

Lesser, M.: NUTRITION AND VITAMIN THERAPY. New York, Grove Press, 1980.

Mindell, E.: VITAMIN BIBLE. New York, Warner Books, 1979.

Montagu, A.: TOUCHING: THE HUMAN SIGNIFICANCE OF THE SKIN. New York, Harper & Row 1972.

Newbold, H.L.: MEGA-NUTRIENTS FOR YOUR NERVES. New York, Wyden Books, 1978.

OUR BODIES, OURSELVES. The Boston Women's Health Book Collective, 465 Mount Auburn Street, Watertown, Maine 02172

Ott, J.N.: HEALTH AND LIGHT. New York, Pocket Books, 1976.

Passwater, R.A.: EVENING PRIMROSE OIL. New Canaan, CT., Keats Publishing, Inc., 1981.

Pfeiffer, C.C.: MENTAL AND ELEMENTAL NUTRIENTS. New Canaan, CT., Keats Publishing, Inc., 1975.

Pfeiffer, C.C.: ZINC AND OTHER MICRO-NUTRIENTS. New Canaan, CT., Keats Publishing, Inc., 1978.

Price, W.A.: NUTRITION AND PHYSICAL DEGENERATION. Price-Pottenger Foundation, P.O. Box 2614, La Mesa, Ca. 92014. 1983 (latest edition).

Schauss, A.: DIET, CRIME AND DELINQUENCY. Berkeley, Ca., Parker House, 1981.

Schroeder, H.A.: THE POISONS AROUND US (Toxic Metals in Food, Air and Water). Bloomington, Ind., University Press, 1974.

Schroeder, H.A.: TRACE ELEMENTS AND MAN, Old Greenwich, CL., Devon-Adair.

Sheinkin, D., Schacter, M. and Hutton, R.: FOOD, MIND & MOOD. New York, Warner Books, 1980.

Sloan, S.: NUTRITIONAL PARENTING. New Canaan, Connecticut, Keats Publishing, Inc., 1982.

Smith, L.H.: FEED YOUR KIDS RIGHT. New York, McGraw-Hill, 1979.

Smith, L.H.: FOODS FOR HEALTHY KIDS. New York, McGraw-Hill, 1981.

Stevens, L. J.: THE NEW WAY TO SUGAR FREE COOKING. New York, Doubleday (publication date August, 1984).

THE WOMANLY ART OF BREAST FEEDING. Franklin Park, Ill., La Leche League, International, 1981.

Williams, R.J.: NUTRITION AGAINST DISEASE. New York, Bantam Books, 1973.

Williams, R.J.: PHYSICIAN'S HANDBOOK OF NUTRITIONAL SCIENCE. Springfield, Illinois, Charles C. Thomas, 1975.

Williams, R.J.: A PHYSICIAN'S HANDBOOK ON ORTHO-MOLECULAR MEDICINE. Elmsford, New York, Pergamon Press, 1977.

Wolf, R. (ed.): EATING BETTER FOR LESS: A GUIDE TO MANAGING YOUR PERSONAL FOOD SUPPLY. Emmaus, Pa., Rodale Press, 1978.

Wright, J.V.: DR. WRIGHT'S BOOK OF NUTRITIONAL THERAPY. Emmaus, Pa., Rodale Press, 1979.

Wunderlich, R.C., Jr.: SUGAR AND YOUR HEALTH. St. Petersburg, Fla., Good Health Publications, Johnny Reads, Inc., 1982.

Index

A

Abdominal pain, 12, 24, 70, 128, 134, 179, 183, 185, 193, 194
Abplanalp, Judith M., 187, 188
Abraham, Guy E., 290
Accent®, 77
Access To Nutritional Data, 261
Aching, 182, 183
Acidophilus (see also *Lactobacillus Acidophilus* and milk, sweet acidophilus)
Acne, 17, 30, 60, 194, 214-215
Addiction, food, 128
Adverse reaction to foods, 87 (see also allergies, food)
Adenoids, enlarged, 203
AIDS, 12, 13
Alcoholic beverages, 70, 77, 90
    craving for, a symptom in yeast-connected illness, 31, 190, 194
Allergic shiners, 6, 128, 206
Allergies, 144, 147, 149
    food, 13, 43, 50, 52, 87, 119, 127-130, 146, 253, 265
        addiction, 128
        controversy over, 253
        hidden, 43, 128, 243
        methods of testing and treating, 253
        obvious, 128
        rotated diets, 128-130, 265

treatment of with allergy extracts, 253
    inhalant, 13, 43, 52, 146
Allergists
    American College of 253
    different methods of testing used by various allergy groups, 253
Allergy
    vaccines (see Immunotherapy or Extracts)
Allergy Alert (a newsletter), 261
Allergy Information Association (Canada), 261
Allergy Shot (a Canadian periodical), 261
Alling, D. W., 256
Alternative health care, 267-269
    controvery over, 268
Alternative medicine,
    as a growth industry in Britain, 268
    Journal of, 269
Amalgam/Mercury toxicity (see Mercury/Amalgam toxicity)
American Academy of Allergy and Immunology, 253
American Academy of Pediatrics, 90, 203
American Academy of Otolaryngic Allergy, 203, 253
American Cyanamid Company, 44, 210
American Medical News, 269
American Pharmacy (magazine), 292

315

Amino acids, 137, 164-165, 292-293
tests for
Amphotericin B, 50, 235, 236,
279-282, 292
prolonged oral treatment with,
safety of, 280-281
use in treating yeast-connected
illness, 280-282
Ampicillin, 30, 59, 78, 201
Amoxicillin, 30, 59, 78, 205
Anah, C., 166
Anatomy of an Illness, (a book by
Norman Cousins) 166, 244, 257
Annals of Allergy, 283, 284
Antibiotic, antibiotics, xv, xvi, 11, 14,
15, 17, 18, 42, 78, 198
broad spectrum, 14
relationship to yeast-connected
illness 17, 18
in anxiety & depression, 224, 225
in multiple sclerosis, 221, 222,
225
in rheumatoid arthritis, 223, 224
in schizophrenia, 225
in teenagers, 213-215
role in promoting yeast growth,
and yeast-connected illness,
x, xvi, 6, 14, 15, 17, 30, 59-60,
190, 214-215, 221-223
therapy of acne, 215
promotes yeast-connected
illness, 17, 30, 60, 90
Antibodies, 9, 164, 286
Antioxidants,
role in protection against free
radical pathology, 285
Anxiety, 129, 183, 185, 187, 193, 214
Aquarian Conspiracy, The (a book by
Marilyn Ferguson) 262, 269-270
Arizona Department of Public
Health, 295
Arthritis, 3, 12, 58, 134, 180, 188
Ascorbate (see vitamin C)
Aspartame, 123-124, 295-296 (see also
Equal®)

Asthma, 168, 184, 185
use of nystatin in therapy, 245
use of vitamin C in therapy, 166,
244-245
Athlete's foot, 23, 28, 40, 173, 194
Attention deficit disorder, 168 (see
also Hyperactivity)
Attention span (short), 213, 214
Autism,
relationship to candida, 195-197,
289-290

B

B-cells, 143, 288
Backache, 187
Bactrim® , 30, 59, 78, 200-201
Baker, Sidney M., iii, 165, 167, 168,
174
Bakery products, 41
Bananas, 75, 79, 80, 82, 97
as trigger of symptoms,
in multiple sclerosis, 124
in multiple sclerosis, 124
Barkie, Karen, 93, 124, 296
Barnes, Broda, 252
Basement,
role in triggering symptoms, 57,
252
Bestways Magazine, 121, 299
Beta carotene, 285
Beverages
alcoholic, 31, 77, 90
beer, 77, 90, 217
as trigger in causing symptoms in
yeast-connected illness, 26
promotes yeast growth in
teenagers, 215
diet drinks, 90
fruit juices, 78, 89
milk, 100, 118, 119, 293-294
water, 86, 90-91
Bible, 127, 234
Billings, F. Tremaine, 258

Biocenter Laboratories, 287
Bionostics, Inc., 287, 292
Bioscience Laboratories, 287
Birmingham Symposium, *The Yeast-Human Interaction-1983*, 274, 275, 288
Birth control pills, xvi, 14, 15, 19, 36, 58, 60, 161, 184, 214-215, 233, 237, 291
  adverse reactions to (see intolerance to)
  avoidance of,
    in treating yeast-connected illness, 36, 268
  intolerance to, a clue in diagnosing yeast-connected illness, 188
  possible role in yeast-connected illness, 179, 184, 185, 190
  role in promoting yeast growth, 14, 15, 179, 190
Blackout, blackouts,
  in nutrition education, 298
  in yeast-connected illness, 159
Bladder,
  infections (see Urinary tract, infections of)
  symptoms (see Urinary tract, problems of)
Bland, Jeffrey, 261, 309
Bloating, 6, 24, 39, 70, 134, 187, 194, 290
Bluestone, Charles D., 204
Body Is The Hero, The (book by Ronald T. Glasser), 164, 166
Bolton, Sanford, 292
Bowel tolerance test,
  use in determining dose of vitamin C, 244-245, 278
Bradley, Cecil, 197
Brain, 174 (see also Nervousness)
  relationship to immune system, and the endocrine system, 174
Brain/Mind Bulletin, 262
Braun, Bob, 271
Breads, 41, 73, 92

yeast-free, 43, 86
Breakfast
  ideas for, 121
  meal suggestions 79-80, 101-102
  Candida Control Diet, 79-80
  Low Carbohydrate Diet, 101-102
  7-day meal plan, 107-110
Breasts, 291
  small, 178, 179, 188
  soreness or pain, 6, 187
Breathing difficulty, 159
Brewer, Tom, 299
Bridges, Turner, 68, 69
British Holistic Medical Association, 268
British Journal of Dermatology, 289
Brodsky, James, 180, 181, 277
Brody, Jane, 69, 312
Bronchial, infections (see Bronchitis)
Bronchitis, 14, 18, 183, 188
Bullock, J.D., 208
Bursitis, 188

C

Cable News Network, 271
Calcium and magnesium
  deficiencies, 88
  supplements, 6, 138, 246, 299
Camel (illustration), 14
Campbell, Don S., 197, 229, 289
Canadian Schizophrenia Foundation, 262
Cancer, 12
Canada,
  Allergy Information Association of, 261
  En-Trophy Institute of, 263
  Human Ecology Foundation of, 263
Candida albicans, 2, 3, 55, 56, 283
  cultures of, 248
  relation to other yeasts and molds, 272, 283

suspected role in causing illness, 17-26

Symposium on, Candida Infections, (book by H. I. Winner and R. Hurley), 283

transmission of,
  through non-sexual contacts, 40, 252
  through sexual relations, 40, 252

Candida and Candidosis (book by F. C. Odds), 255

Candida Conference,
  Birmingham, 274-275
  Dallas, xv, 91, 199, 226, 261-264

Candida Control Diet, 72, 73, 75-93, 266, 293
  Additional Helpful Suggestions, 87-93
  Foods You Can Eat, 75-76
  Foods You Must Avoid, 77-78
  Food Sources, 86
  Meal Suggestions, 79-84
  Shopping Tips, 85

Candida krusei, 283

Candida tropicalis, 283

Candidiasis (see Yeast-connected illness)
  chronic mucocutaneous, 4, 248

Carbohydrates,
  complex, 42, 67-70, 95, 117-118, 137
  contributions to good health, vii, 67-70, 73, 95
  good, (see Carbohydrates, complex)
  Low Carbohydrate Diet, 69, 70, 73, 95-110
  not to be limited in children, 43
  relationship to yeast growth, 42, 70-71, 119

Carbohydrate-free soy formula (RCF)® , 209

Carlson, Eunice, 275

CAT Scan, 159

Cathcart, R. F., iii, 244

Cave Man Diet, 243

improvement on, 196, 277

Ceclor® , 18, 30, 59, 78, 184, 185

Cellar (see Basement)

Center for Early Education of Handicapped, 197

Center for Science in the Public Interest (CSPI), 260, 299

Cereal grains, (see also grains) 43, 76, 91

Chemicals,
  avoiding, 150, 210, 250, 267
  barrel concept (illustration), 156-157
  environmental, 13, 152-157, 159-162
  how they cause illness, 157
  illness due to, v, vi, 3, 6, 12, 20, 61, 149, 150, 151, 160, 161, 185, 191, 192, 193, 294, 295
    treatment with antioxidants, 285
    treatment with nystatin and diet, 159-62
    treatment with immunotherapy, 298
  offenders, 152-155
  sensitivity & susceptibility to, xv, 12
    lessens with anti-candida treatment, 159-162, 273
    managing, 153, 210
    relationship to *Candida albicans,* 20, 159-162
    use of selenium, vitamin C and other antioxidants in treatment, 285
    weaken immune system, 13

Cheraskin, E., 67, 167, 208

Chest pain, 5, 25, 68, 183

Children, 42, 43
  diet in, 43
  ear infections in (see Ear, Problems and Infections)
  yeast-connected illness in, 42, 43, 195-211 (see also Yeast-connected Illness, in children)

Christie, Amos U., iii, 258

Chronic mucocutaneous candidiasis, 4, 248
Cleveland, Ohio, support groups, 260
Clinical ecologists, 251
Clinical Ecology,
    organizations and publications relating to, 259-264
    physicians who practice, 277
    Seminar, November, 1983, 283
    Society for, 4, 203, 253
    textbook, *Clinical Ecology* edited by Lawrence Dickey, M.D., 309
Clotrimazole, use in oral and vaginal candidiasis, 256
Codeine,
    adverse effects of, 6
Coffee, 78, 90
Cohen and associates, 248
Colic, 195, 202, 203
    treatment with nystatin, 202-203
Colitis, ulcerative, 168, 180 (see also Crohn's disease)
Colon,
    irritable, 129
    spastic, 237
Complementary medicine, 268
Concentrate, inability to, 21, 202
Condiments, 77, 91
Conference, Dallas (see Dallas Candida Conference)
Connolly, Pat, 119, 293
Constipation, 24, 28, 39, 175, 179, 194
    persistent,
    use of nystatin enemas in treatment, 248-249
Consumer,
    information and organizations, 259-262, 298-300
Consumer Reports (publication), 91
Consumerism,
    in medicine, 268-270
Cooper, Max, 274, 280, 283
Corn syrup,
    as a triggering factor in

    hyperactivity, 67
Corticosteroids, xiv, 20, 233
Cortisone, 20
Cosmopolitan (magazine), 291, 299
Cough, 3, 25, 160, 184
Cousins, Norman, 166, 244, 257, 258, 269
Crackers, yeast-free, 43
Cranton, Elmer, iii, 71, 285, 287, 297
Cravings, 191
Creative Audio, 275
Critical Illness Research Foundation, ix, 302
Crohn's disease, 168, 218, 226
Crying Baby, Sleepless Nights (book by Sandy Jones), 203
Curlin, John, 100, 202, 207, 277
Cutis (publication), 4
Cystitis, 182 (see Urinary Infections)
Cytotoxic food test, 71

D

Dallas Candida Conference, xv, 91, 199, 226, 271-275
Dalton, Katharina, 187
Damp, dampness,
    as promoter of mold growth, 55
    as trigger of symptoms, 57, 58, 194
    in yeast-connected illness, 26
    measures to overcome, 55, 56
Damp Chaser Electronics, 56
Daniel, Book of, 127
Davey, Paula, 251
Davis, Donald R., 255
Davis, Rebecca, iii, 73
Deamer, W. C., iii, 208, 258
Depression 12, 21
    as manifestation of amino acid disorder, 292, 293
    as manifestation of inhaled mold, 58, 58
    as manifestation of yeast-connected illness, v, vi, 12, 21, 46, 57, 58,

129, 135, 149, 152, 159, 171,
178, 180, 185, 187, 188, 192,
193, 194, 202, 213, 214, 234,
248, 294
as a reaction to nystatin, 46
as a reaction to sugar, 88
provoked by candida extract, 58
Diabetes, 68
Diagnosis of yeast-connected illness
(see Yeast-connected illness,
diagnosis of)
Diaper rashes,
persistent, relation to antibiotics,
252
Diarrhea, 24, 39, 194
Dickey Enterprises, 130
Dickey, Lawrence, iii, 272, 277, 309
Die-off symptoms, from nystatin, 45,
249
Diets,
Candida Control (see also Candida
Control Diet), 75-93, 266, 293
during pregnancy, 299
Fruit-Free, Sugar-Free, Yeast-Free,
73, 117, 265, 266
Fruit-Free, Grain-Free, Nut-Free,
Milk-Free, Yeast-Free,
Sugar-Free, 73, 119, 265
good diet, 52
high carbohydrate, 68
role in heart disease, prevention
and treatment, 68
low carbohydrate (see also Low
Carbohydrate Diet), viii, 50, 69,
72, 95-110, 243, 266, 272, 277,
280, 293
rotated, 130, 243, 300
teenage, 216, 217
twentieth century, 14, 15
Digestive,
enzymes, 256
problems, 191, 248 (see also specific
symptoms, e.g., constipation,
bloating, etc.)
Dilantin® , 159

Diseases,
labelling of, 167-172
Divorce,
relation to candida, 180, 181, 291
Dizziness, 3, 58, 160, 182, 193
Doctor's Data (a laboratory), 287
Donahue, Phil, 216
Drained, 21, 193
Drowsiness, 22, 127
Dr. Mandell's 5-Day Allergy Relief
System, (book), 61
"Drunk disease", 197, 229-230
Drunkenness,
related to candida, 197, 229-230,
Dry Bones, 173

E

Ear,
pain in, 3
problems and infections, 18, 42, 59,
183, 195, 196, 203-211
use of nystatin along with
antibiotics, 59, 206-208, 210
ringing in (tinnitus), 173
suggestions for management in
infants, 208-211
tubes, 203-303, 213
Eating out, 93, 120
Ecology (see Clinical Ecology)
Ecology Society (British), 264
EEG studies, 134
Efamol® , (see Fatty Acids, primrose
oil)
Elman, Suzi, 271
Emotional disorders, 159, 186, 187
(see also Nervousness,
Hyperactivity)
role of refined carbohydrates in
promoting, 67
Endocrine system (see also
Hormone, hormones)
relations to candida, 174

relation to immune system, 174
Endometriosis, 180
Enemas,
    cortisone, 249
    nystatin, 235, 249
England,
    alternative health care,
        discussion of, 268-269
        listing of groups and facilities,
        264
En-Trophy Institute of Canada, 263
Enzymes, digestive, 256
Environmental Health Association of
    Dallas, 260
Epidermophyton,
    immunotherapy, 278
EPO (Evening primrose oil), 246
Equal® , 73, 123, 124 (see also
    aspartame)
Erratic behavior, (see also
    Hyperactivity), 213
Erythromycin, 59
    less apt to promote growth of
        candida, 59
Essential fatty acids (see Fatty Acids,
    Essential)
Evening primrose oil (see Primrose
    Oil, fatty acids)
Executive Health, 246, 262, 298
Exercise, 105, 110, 111, 146, 267,
    294 295
    importance of,
        in overcoming yeast-connected
            illness, 135, 294-295
        in promoting good health, 135,
            143, 144, 146, 148
Extract, candida, 37 (see also
    Immunotherapy)
    as cause of depression, 58
Eye problems, 32, 33, 222
    blurring, 25
    burning, 33, 157, 193
    spots in front of, 25, 32
    tearing, 33
    visual difficulty, 33, 233

F

Family,
    treatment of, in patients with
        yeast-connected illness, 252
Family Circle (magazine), 229
Fatigue, v, vi, 6, 12, 21, 28, 45, 46, 58,
    70, 127, 129, 135, 149, 159, 171,
    175, 178, 179, 182, 184, 185, 188,
    192, 194, 223, 232, 236, 248
    as manifestation of amino acid
        disorder, 292
Fatty acids, essential, 135, 138, 141,
    148, 150, 152, 246, 288
    use of,
        in multiple sclerosis, 13, 220, 221,
            223, 267
        in premenstrual syndrome, 188,
            228, 290
FDA (see Food & Drug
    Administration)
Females,
    susceptibility to yeast-connected
        illness,
    reasons for, 188-190
Ferguson, Marilyn, 269
Fields, I., 251
Flora, Betty, iii, 70
Flu-like symptoms, 45 (see also
    Nystatin, die-off symptoms)
Food, Foods, (see Diet, Grains, etc.)
    allergic-like reactions caused by
        amino acids abnormalities, 292
    cleaning of with Clorox® , 256, 257
    chemically contaminated, 152, 153
    fabricated, 69
    processed, 69
    sources, 86
Food allergies (see Allergies, food)
Food & Drug Administration, 123,
    230, 292
Formaldehyde, xv, 152, 160
    contamination of home, 196
    use in controlling molds in the
        home, 61-64

Formalin (see Formaldehyde)
Free radicals, 285
  nature of, 285
  pathology from, 285
  protective role of antioxidants, 285
  role in causing chemical
    hypersensitivity, 285
Freeman Report, 271
Freeman, Sandi, 271
Fructose, 123, 125
Fruits, 70, 75, 77, 124
  as a cause of symptoms, 70, 119
  role in promoting good health, vii,
    67-69
  role in promoting yeast growth,
    viii, 42, 43, 117-119, 125, 255,
    300
Fruit-Free, Sugar-Free, Yeast-Free
  Diet, 73, 117-118, 266
Fruit-Free, Yeast-Free, Sugar-Free,
  Grain-Free, Nut-Free, Milk-Free
  Diet, 73, 119
Fruit juices, 78, 89
Frustration, 146, 148
Fungizone® , 280
  (see also Amphotericin B)
Fungus, Fungi (see also Athlete's
  foot, Jock itch, Molds and Yeasts)
  of skin, 12
  of nails, 12, 192
Furadantin® ,
  use in urinary tract infections, 60,
    201

G

Galen, 3
Galland, Leo, 275
Gallstones, 134
Galton, Lawrence, 252
Gamma globulin (see IgA, IgE, etc)
Garlic, 25, 267, 291-292
Gas (see also Bloating, Digestive
  problems)
Gas heat, (see Chemicals)

Gastritis, 193
Gastro-intestinal (see Digestive
  problems)
Germs,
  friendly, 10, 11
  yeast, 10, 11
Gerdes, Ken, 277, 297
Gerrard, John W., iii, 208
Gesell Institute of Human
  Development, iii, 165, 275
Glasser, Ronald T., 163, 164, 166
Glucose tolerance test, 182, 237
Glutathione, 285
Gluten, 70, 71 (see also grains)
Goodman and Gilman,
  *Pharmocological Basis of
  Therapeutics*, (book), 281
Grains, 42, 67, 69, 70, 91, 92, 98, 99
  do they promote yeast growth?
  no, viii, 42
  yes, vii, 70
  induced reactions, 70, 255
  whole, 67, 69, 70, 85
  use on low carbohydrate diet,
    101-110
  source of, 86

H

Hagglund, Howard, 277
Hair analysis, 285
Hall, Judy, 260
Hall, Ross Hume, 69
Handwriting, altered, 187
Hardy, James F., 297
Hayfever, 183
Headache, vi, 3, 12, 21, 45, 46, 57, 58,
    129, 134, 149, 157, 159, 160, 171,
    173, 175, 178, 179, 183, 183, 186,
    188, 192, 193, 213, 214, 223, 237,
    281, 294
Healing Heart, The (a book by Norman
  Cousins), 257, 258, 269
Healing resources,

mobilizing of, 257-258
Health Guidance Center (Cleveland, Ohio), 262
Hearing loss, 203
Heart,
    disease, 68
    heartburn, 24
    palpitations, 151, 159
    rapid (tachycardia), 237
Hedges, Harold, 128, 129, 277
Helper cells, 286
Helper/Suppressor ratio, 286
Henderson, John A., 119, 293-294
Herman, Daniel A., 251
Herxheimer reactions, 45 (see also Nystatin "die-off" symptoms)
Hilsheimer, George Von, 266
Hippocrates, 3, 127, 291
Hives,
    yeast-connected, v, 149, 192, 193, 288-289
Hoffman-LaRoche, 230
Hofstra & associates, 248
Holistic medicine, 268, 269 (see also alternative medicine)
Hollister-Stier Laboratories, 63
Honey, 41, 124-125
    promotes yeast growth, viii, 42, 43, 71
Hormone, (see also Endocrine)
    changes, 14, 15, 179, 189, 190, 291
    imbalances, 190, 251-252
    poor function, 175, 225
    improvement in function with anti-candida therapy, 175
Horrobin, David, 141, 246, 290
Hospital Practice (publication), 187
House,
    moldy, role in triggering symptoms, 57, 58, 252
Huggins, Hal, 296, 297
Human Ecology Action League (HEAL), 259
Human Ecology Foundation of Canada, 262

Human Ecologist, 265
Humidifiers,
    encourage mold growth, 57
Hunter, Beatrice Trum, 69
Huxley Institute of Biosocial Research, 198, 262
Huxley, Thomas, xx
Hyperactive Children's Support Group (English), 264
Hyperactivity, 42, 67, 125, 129, 134, 195-198, 201, 202, 205, 206 (see also Yeast-connected Illness, Symptoms of, in children)
    sugar and, 67, 125, 196-200
Hypochondriasis, 129, 189
Hypoglycemia, 182, 237
Hypothyroidism, 252
Hysterectomy, 185, 235

I

Idiosyncracy, food, 127 (see also Allergies, food)
IgA (Gammaglobulin A), 9,
IgG (Gammaglobulin G), 9,
Illness,
    causes of,
        multiple factors play a role, 51, 131-176
Immune system, xv, 8-15, 52, 142, 143, 163-166, 183
    factors which weaken, 13, 165, 179, 191, 210
    how it protects you, 163, 166
    relationship to brain & nervous symptoms, 174, 179, 191
    relationship to candida, 174
    relationship to endocrine system, 174, 175, 179, 191
    strengthening,
        by avoiding pollutants, 267, 295
        by stopping smoking, 267
        through love, touch, faith, hope and prayer, 267, 295

with exercise, 267, 294, 295
with lifestyle changes, 267
with nutritional supplements, 267, 295
with vitamin C, 210, 245
Immunoglobulins, 9
Immunotherapy, 150, 172, 174, 252-255, 273, 277
   candida, 37, 273
   requires careful monitoring, 273
   chemical, 254, 278-279
   food, 254, 278-279
   hormone, 254
   inhalant, 254, 278-279
   methods of administering,
      "build-up", 253, 273
      Miller, 253
      provocative/neutralization technique, 253, 273
      Rinkel, 253
      serial dilution technique, 193, 253, 273-274, 278-279
   TOE (TCE . . . combined extract of trichophyton, candida and epidermophyton), 278
Immune complexes, 8, 10
Immunodiagnostic Laboratory
Impotence, 31 (see also Sex and Sexual)
Incoordination, 22, 174, 182, 187, 202
Index Medicus, 291
Indigestion, 24 (see also bloating, digestive problems, etc.)
Infection, 14, 15
   bacterial, 12, 142
   ear, 18
   urinary, 18
   viral, 12, 142
Infertility, 178, 180, 181, 188
Information,
   Other Sources of, 258-264, 265
Inhalant allergies (see Allergies, Inhalant)
Insomnia, 186, 207
Insta-Tape, Inc., 261

Intestinal tract, 10, 11
Intercourse, sexual,
   in teenagers, 216
   painful, 178, 180, 188
International Journal of Biosocial Research, 263
Ionizers, air, 255
Iron,
   deficiency, 138
   supplements of, 246
Irrational behavior, 186
Irritability, 21, 40, 43, 67, 149, 159, 160, 178, 180, 188, 192, 198, 207
   related to sugar, 88
   response to nystatin, 202
Iwata, Kazuo, 197, 230, 275

J

Jackson Sun, The, 58, 213
Jane Brody's Nutrition Book, 69, 312
Jock itch, 23, 40, 194
Joints,
   pain in, vi, 3, 128, 151, 157, 186, 192, 223, 236, 354
   swelling of, 3, 58 (see also Arthritis)
Johns Hopkins University, 166
Johnson, Jim, 265
Jones, Sandy, 203
Journal of Allergy and Clinical Immunology, 210
Journal of American College of Nutrition, 290
Journal, the International, of Biosocial Research, 263
Journal of Orthomolecular Psychiatry, 4, 13, 198, 259, 262, 266, 271, 285
Journal of the American Medical Association, 253
Journal of Reproductive Medicine, 290

K

Keats Publishing Co., 246, 285

Keflex® , 18, 30, 59, 78, 184, 185, 237
Keough, Carol, 91
Ketoconazole (see Nizoral®)
Kidney infections, 59 (see also Urinary tract)
Kirkpatrick, Charles H. 248, 256
Kitchen,
  chemicals in, 155
  role in triggering symptoms, 57
Kupsinel, Roy, 263, 297
Kup's Komments (newsletter), 263
Kroker, George, 263, 277

L

Labelling diseases, 167-171
Laboratory studies,
  in patients with yeast-connected illness, 285-288
    amino acid studies, 287
    blood vitamin studies, 287
    fatty acid studies, 288
    immune system studies, 286
      antibody studies, 286-287
      helper/suppressor ratio, 286
      T-cell studies, 286
    mineral studies, 287
Lactobacillus Acidophilus,
  deficiency of in stools,
    in psychiatric patients, 266
    in patients with gastrointestinal symptoms, 266
  supplementation with,
    freeze-dried capsules, 267
    sweet acidophilus milk, 267
    yogurt, 267
Lactose (see also milk),
  in milk, 100
    promotes candida growth, 293-294
Ladies Home Journal (magazine), 299
Landers, Ann, 216
La Pachol (see Taheebo tea)

Lay support group (see Support Group)
Learning problems (see also Yeast-connected illness, in children)
  as manifestation of amino acid disorder, 292
  in children with yeast connected illness, 195-197
Lederle Laboratories, 44, 210
Lee, Carlton, 253
Leftovers, 77, 91
Lemon juice,
  salad dressing in combination with oil, 85
Lethargy, lethargic, 21 (see also Fatigue and Depression)
Let's Live (magazine), 299
Levin, Alan, ix, 197, 295
Levine, Steven A., 285
Lewis, Don, 277
Libido, loss of (see Sex, Sexual)
Lidocaine® ,
  adverse reactions to, 6
Lieberman, Allan, iii, 202, 277
Lind, James, 71
Lingo, John, 133
Linseed oil, 85, 150, 155, 172, 221, 246, 267 (see also Fatty acids, essential)
Lister, John, 268
Liver
  function tests
    in patients taking Nizoral® , 49, 192
  toxicity
    in patients taking Nizoral® 48-49
    no serious reactions seen by physicians, 278
London, Robert S., 290
London Times, The, 264
Long Island Pediatrician, 90
Lorenzani, Shirley, 71, 119, 293
Lorimer, Janet, 121

Los Angeles Times, 197, 229-230
Low Carbohydrate Diet, viii, 69, 72,
    95-100, 243, 266, 272
    Foods You Can Eat Freely, 95-97
    Foods You Can Eat Cautiously,
      97-100
    Meal Suggestions, 101-106
    7-Day Meal Plan, 107-110
Lown, Bernard, 257
Lucas, Patricia, 40, 252
Lucretius, 127
Lupus erythematosus, systemic, 168

M

MS (see Multiple Sclerosis)
Mabray, Richard, 180, 188, 277
Maclennan, John, iii, 262
Macrodantin® , 60, 201
Mandell, Marshall, iii, 61-64
Marital
    difficulties, 185, 186, 291
      relationship to candida, 180, 181,
        291
    partner
      treatment of, 40, 252
May, Charles, 257
Mayer, Jean, 298
Mayo, Duffy, 197
McCarrison Society, The, 264
Medical care
    high cost of, vi, 172, 268
Medication,
    for yeast-connected illness, 44-50,
      277-278 (see also Nystatin,
      Nizoral® , Amphotericin B,
      Clotrimazole)
Medicine,
    alternative, 267-268
    complementary, 268
    consumerism, in, 268
    orthodox, 268

Megatrends, (a book by John Naisbitt),
    270
Memory loss, 39, 58, 174, 182, 184,
    248
Men,
    health problems of, 191-194
Mendelsohn, Robert, 263
Menstrual, menstruation,
    cramps, viii, 32, 39, 175, 180, 181,
      182, 183, 184, 185, 216, 232
    irregularities, viii, 23, 32, 39, 173,
      178, 179, 180, 194 (see also
      PMS)
Mental confusion, 58, 149, 193
    caused by exposure to tobacco
      smoke, 193
Mental disease, (see also
    Depression)
    related to candida, 213-214,
      218,-219, 289
Mental dullness, 58, 127
Mercury/amalgam toxicity, 296-297
Metabolic Update (audio tape), 261
Metabolism disorders, 293
Metei-sho (Japanese "drunk
    disease"), 197, 229-230
Migraine, 58, 168, 179, 233 (see also
    Headache)
Milk,
    lactose in,
      promotes yeast growth, 76, 100,
        293-294
      sweet acidophilus, 100, 266-267
Miller, Joseph, iii, 180, 253
MineraLab, 287
Minerals, 165
    trace, 259, 285, 299
Missing Diagnosis, The, vii, 4, 167,
    201, 207, 259, 265
Mitchell, George, 277
Mittelman, Jerome, 263, 296-297
Mittelman Newsletter, 297
Molds, 2, 55-64, 87, 89, 91
    affect immune system, xvi

avoidance of, 51, 89, 250
characteristics of, 55-56
controlling yeasts & molds, 57-64
  avoid antibiotics, 59
  avoid 'the pill', 60-61
cultures of, 63, 283-285
  lack of accuracy in older
      methods, 283-284
  new methods, 283-285
illustrations of, 2, 54
in bathtub, 36
in diet,
  comments on 89-94, 118
inhalation of,
  as a cause of depression, 57-58
  as a cause of other symptoms,
      58-59
relationship to yeasts, 55
sources of, 55-64
  in homes, 36, 51, 56-57
survey service, 284
treatment with formaldehyde
    vapors, 61-64
Mold Survey Service, 283-285
Monilia albicans, 3 (see also Yeasts &
    Candida Albicans)
Monistat® , vaginal suppositories or
    cream
Monroe Medical Laboratories, 287
Montes, Leopoldo, 280-283
Mood swings, 182, 185
Mould (see Molds)
Multiple sclerosis, vi, 12, 124, 134,
    168, 218-227
  relationship to *candida albicans*
      218-227
Muscle aches, 128, 184
Muscle weakness, 220-226
Mushrooms,
  adverse reactions to, 196
Myasthenia gravis, 218
Mycostatin® , 44 (see also nystatin)
Mycelex G® , vaginal cream, 247
Mysteclin-F® , 279

N

Naisbitt, John, 270
Narcolepsy, 182
Nasal, (see also nose)
  congestion, 6, 25, 43, 128, 184, 185,
      192, 193, 200, 206, 248, 281
  relief obtained with intranasal
      nystatin, 202, 248
  infection, 14
National Academy of Sciences,
  Food and Nutrition Board
  dietary recommendations, 67
National Cancer Institute, 251
National Women's Health Network,
  260
Nausea, 3, 159, 186
Nervous breakdown, 58
Nervousness, 12, 21, 39, 67, 159, 160,
    182, 191, 192, 194
Neurological disease,
  yeast-connected, 218-227
Neurosis,
  as manifestation of amino acid
      disorder, 292
New England Journal of Medicine, 204,
    227, 267, 269, 299
New Jersey, Medical College of, 234
New Woman (publication), 298
Nilstat® , 44 (see also nystatin)
Nizoral® , vii, 235, 238, 239, 272, 278,
    289
  adverse reactions, 48-49, 235
  cost of, 50
  indications for use, 48-50
  liver function tests prior to use, 49
  successful use of, 272, 278, 282
  use in combination with nystatin,
      278
Norwich Eaton Pharmaceuticals,
    Inc., 201
Nose,
  Congestion of, (see Nasal
      congestion)

Null, Gary, 292
Numbness, 22, 124, 220, 222, 223
Nutra, Sara Sloan, 261
Nutrasweet® (see also Aspartame),
   123
Nutrition, (see also Foods, Diet, Fatty
   acids, Vitamins)
  education, blackout in, 297
  good,
    for teenagers, 217
    importance of, 67-69, 135,
      137-141, 144-145
  poor,
    In teenagers, 216
    sources of good food, 67-69,
      137-139
    sources of information, 297-298
Nutrition Action, (publication), 265
Nutrition for Optimal Health Association
   (NOHA), 260
Nutritional deficiencies, 13
  role in causing yeast-connected
    illness, 219
Nutritional supplements, 149, 188,
   220, (see also Vitamins, Fatty
   Acids)
  use of by physicians, 278
Nuts, 86, 92, 94, 97
  possible mold contamination of, 78,
    85, 119
  unprocessed, source of, 86
Nystatin, 35, 44-47, 272, 273
  absorption of, 45
  adverse reactions (side effects), 45,
    46, 249
  cost of, 47, 50
  die-off symptoms, 45, 185, 249, 272
  dosage, 44, 45, 48, 49, 249
    "dot dose", 46
    larger dose needed to obtain
      good response, 277-278
  duration of therapy, 48, 273
  dye-free capsules, 48
  enemas, 235, 248
  favorable response, to, 6, 182, 186

    (see also yeast-connected
     illness, treatment of)
  foot powder, 44
  intranasal, 247, 248
  intravaginal, 44, 247
  mechanism of action, 249
  powder, 44-47
  prophylactic use,
    in infants of children, 59, 198,
      199, 210
    in adults, 59
  safety of, 44, 50
  sniffing of, powder, 247
  tablets, 44, 45, 47
  therapy in,
    asthma, 245
    infants & children, 196, 202, 206,
      207, 210
    teenagers, 213-214
    men, 192-194
    multiple sclerosis, 219-227
    women, 179-188
  underdose symptoms, 46
  use by different physicians,
    272-273, 277-278
  use of,
    as anti-fungal medication, 35, 281
    in severe asthma, 244-245

O

Oberg, Gary, 227
Odds, F. C., M.D., 4, 43, 255, 271
Odium albicans, 3 (see also *Candida
   albicans*)
Ohishi, Kozo, 229
Omega Tech Laboratory, 287
Once Daily (a newsletter), 263
Orr, A. Stephens, 188
Orthomolecular (see also *Journal of
   Orthomolecular Psychiatry*)
  explanation of meaning of the
    word, 298
  nutrition, 298

O'Shea, James A., 256, 257, 277
Osler, William, 166
Osteoporosis, 299
Otitis media (see Ear Infections)
Ott, John, 132
Outgassing, 154 (see also Chemical, Chemicals)

P

Pachovich, M. J., 263
Pan American Allergy Society, 253
Pancreatic enzymes,
    breakdown lactose, 293
Pancreatin, 256
Pangborn, John, 292
Paranoid feelings,
    in yeast-connected illness, 294
Passwater, Richard A., 246,
Pau D'Arco (see Taheebo Tea)
Pauling, Linus, 142, 165, 244
Peabody, Francis, 258
Pelvic pain, 178, 180, 188
Penicillin G, and penicillin V, 59
People's Doctor, The, 263
Peoples Medical Society, The, 260
Perfume,
    adverse reactions to, xv, 20, 155,
        156-157, 185
Personality,
    change of,
        response to nystatin, 202
Pfeiffer, Carl, 148
Pharmacological Basics of Therapeutics,
    (book), 258
Physician, physicians
    locating a, 265, 266
    practicing, observations on
        yeast-connected illness, 271-275,
        277-278
Physician's Desk Reference, 44, 167,
    279, 282-283
Pill, the, (see Birth control pills)
Pistey, Warren, 275, 283

Pizza,
    as trigger of symptoms in
        yeast-connected illness, 26, 59
Plants and Cancer, Report on, 251
Pneumonia, 184
Pollutants (see Chemicals)
Pollution,
    barrel concept, 156-157
    chemical, 219
Prayer, 186, 234-235, 257, 295, 298
Predictive Medicine, (book by E.
    Cheraskin), 167
Pregnancy, 15, 19
    nausea and vomiting in, 180
    role in promoting yeast growth, 15,
        30, 194
Prednisone, 20
Premenstrual tension (Premenstrual
    Syndrome . . . PMS), 32, 39, 40,
    134, 175, 178, 179, 180, 181, 185,
    186, 187-190, 216, 225, 252, 288,
    290, 291
    role of candida albicans in causing,
        179, 186-188
    symptoms of, 186-188, 290, 291
    treatment of,
        anticandida therapy, 180-188
        fatty acids, essential, 188, 290
        minerals, 187, 290
        use of thyroid supplements, 252
        vitamins, 290
Prevention (magazine), 246, 299
Preventive Medicine Doctor, The, (a
    pamphlet), 263
Price Pottenger Nutrition
    Foundation, 73, 208, 259, 265
    physician's directory, 265-266
Primrose oil, evening, 150, 236, 246,
    267, 290 (see also Fatty acids,
    essential)
Priority Products, Inc., 251
Pritikin, Nathan, 67
Progesterone,
    minidose therapy, 180
    use in treating PMS, 187

vaginal suppositories, 187
Prostaglandins, 138, 187, 246
Prostatitis, 31, 191, 192
Psoriasis, 12, 134, 168
Psychosis, (see also Schizopherenia)
  as manifestation of amino acid
    deficiency, 292
  relationship to Candida albicans,
    219-226
Putka, Gary, 295
Puzzle (illustration), 148
Pyron, J. W., 296-297

Q

Questions and Answers,
  on overcoming yeast-connected
    illness, 39-52
Questionnaire, 172
  patient's,
    for use in suspecting
      yeast-connected illness,
    long, 29-33
    short, x,
  physician's
    response to, viii, 277-279

R

Radcliffe, Michael J., 264
Randolph, Theron, G., iii, v, 200
Rapp, Doris, iii, 128
Rash, rashes, (see Skin Problems)
RAST test, 128, 208, 253
RCF® (a carbohydrate-free soy
  formula), 209-210
Rea, William, iii, 156, 157
Reader's Digest, 299
Recipes, 111-116
Reed, Mary, 58, 213
Reinhardt, Jeffrey H., 285
Respiratory problems, 14, 42, 184,
  191, 194, 209

treatment of,
  penicillin & erythromycin less
    apt to promote candida
    growth, 59
Revolution, In Medicine, The Coming, vi
Rhinitis, 149, 174, 183, 188 (see also
  Nose, congestion of)
Rice cakes & crackers, 85
  source of, 86
Richardson, Rich, 68
Richardson, Rosemary, 68
Ringsdorf, W. M., Jr., 67, 208
Rinkel, Herbert J., 253
Rippon, J. W., viii, 3, 4, 42, 43, 73, 75,
  89, 94, 117, 118, 251, 275, 294
  transcript of Crook-Rippon
    interview, 117-118
Robley, Cheryl, 135, 185, 186, 213
Rockwell, Sally, 261
Rodale Press, 91
Rogers, Sherry, A., 63, 283-285
Rose, Robert M., 187, 188
Rosenberg, E. W., xx, 226, 227, 275
Ross Laboratories, 209
Rotarian, The, (magazine), 298
Rotated diets, 130, 243, 300
Rudin, Donald O., 141

S

Saccharin, 73, 124
Saifer, Phyllis, 46, 197, 251, 277, 288,
  297
Salad dressing,
  lemon juice & oil, 77, 85
Sanity, (British organization), 264
Sara Sloan, Nutra®, (newsletter), 261
Schaeffer, Nathan, 61
Schizophrenia, 218, 219
  Association,
    of Britain, 264
    of Canada, 262
    of Greater Washington, 262
Schroeder, Henry, 165, 299

Science, (a journal), 298
Seizures, 149
  as manifestation of amino acid
    disorder, 292
Selenium, 165
  recommended daily allowance of,
    285
  role as an antioxidant, 285
Septra® , 18, 30, 59, 78
Sex (see also Sexual),
  activity of teenagers, 216
  drive, impaired, 194
Sexual,
  desire, loss of, 180, 188
  intercourse (see Intercourse,
    sexual)
  interest or drive, impairment of, 19,
    94, 188, 194
  relations,
    role in transmission of candida,
      252
  response,
    impairment or loss of, 6, 173, 179,
      180, 188
Shambaugh, George, 203, 204
Sinus, infections of (see Sinusitis)
Sinusitis, 14, 18, 129, 151, 193
Skin,
  dry, 152
  fungus infections of, 23, 178, 191,
    192
Smoke, tobacco
  as a cause of symptoms, 193
Smoking,
  stopping of,
    importance in strengthening
      immune system, 267
Society for Clinical Ecology (see
  Ecology, Society for)
Sohnle, Peter G., 248
Sore throat (see Throat, sore)
Southern Medical Journal, 298
Soy formula, 43, 208-210
Spaced out feeling, 39, 174, 183
Speck, Marvin L., 266

Speer, Frederic, iii, 208
Spices, 91
Squibb, E. R. & Co., 210, 215, 235,
  279-283
Squibb Institute of Medical Research,
  279
Steroids, (see Corticosteroids,
  Prednisone)
Sterrett, Francis S., 90
Stevens, Laura J., 296, 314
Stiffness, 192
Stomach, nervous, 129 (see also
  Digestive prpblems)
Stomachache, 186, 193
Stone Age Diet (see Cave Man Diet)
Sublingual allergy extracts, 254 (see
  also Immunotherapy)
Sugar,
  as a cause of hyperactivity, 67,
    199-201
    possible mechanisms, 88, 89, 200,
      201
  as a cause of symptoms, 93
    behavior and emotional, 43
    respiratory, 43
  avoidance of, 300
  clinical study, 199-200
  craving, 41, 198, 199
  in bakery products, 43
  in dry cereals, 92
  in processed foods, 69, 85
  role in promoting yeast growth, vii,
    xvi, 14, 15, 35, 42
  substitutes, 123-125
  triggering of symptoms in,
    hyperactivity, 67
    multiple sclerosis, 220
    yeast-connected illness, 6
Sugar-free baby food, 209-210
Sugar-free cooking,
  A New Way to Sugar-Free Cooking (a
    cookbook by Laura Jane
    Stevens featuring aspartame),
    295, 314
  Sweet and Sugar-Free (a cookbook

featuring fruits by Karen
Barke), 93, 124, 296
Sulfa Drugs, (see also Sepra®
Bactrim®)
longterm therapy,
relationship to yeast growth and
multiple sclerosis, 223
Suicide,
thoughts of in yeast-connected
illness, 294
Supplements (see also Fatty acids,
Vitamins and *Lactobacillus
Acidophilus*)
calcium and magnesium, 138, 246
iron, 246-247
multivitamin and mineral, 138, 243,
244
Support groups, 172
lay, 258, 260-263, 267
Suppressor cells, 295
Swaart, Charles, 197, 229-230, 289
Sweets (see also Sugar), 88, 89, 93
Sweet and Sugar Free (a
"Fruit-sweetened Cookbook"),
93, 124, 296
Swelling, 192
Szent Györgi, Albert, 71

T

Tachycardia, 237, 288
T-Cells, 143, 273 (see also Immune
system)
Taheebo tea (see Tea, taheebo)
Tapes, audio, 261, 263, 274-275
informational
on nutrition, 261, 274
on yeast, 263, 274, 275
Tea, 78, 89
herbal, 89
taheebo, 89, 250, 251
Teenagers, 213-217
physical & mental problems of (see
also Yeast-Connected Illness)

Teich, Morton, 198, 207, 277
*Tennessee Medical Association, Journal
of,* 5
Tetracyclines, 17, 60, 181, 190, 201,
214, 279 (see also Antibiotics)
role in promoting candida growth,
17, 20, 201, 214
Throat,
infections of, 14
sore, 3, 28, 159, 193, 237
Trichophyton,
immunotherapy, 278
Thrush, 3, 13, 198, 252
Thyroid,
blood studies, 252
*Hypothyroidism: The Unsuspected
Illness,* (book), 252
deficiency,
detection using basal
temperature determinations,
252
disease, inapparent, 252
supplementation, 175
Time (magazine), 229
Tingling, 22, 193
Tobacco, 157 (see also Smoke,
Smoking)
adverse reactions to, xv, 20
as polluter, 153-155
sensitivity to, 151, 185, 254
TOE (TCE or TME) extract, 272 (see
also Immunotherapy)
Toledo, Ohio, Allergy Management
and Support Group, 260
Tonsils,
removal of, 237
Touch, 143, 148
Toxic Element Research Foundation,
297
Toxins, 11, 13 (see also Yeast, toxins)
yeast, xvi, 11, 13, 15, 164
Tracking Down Hidden Food Allergy,
(book by William Crook), 71, 87,
128, 196, 243
Trace Elements, Hair Analysis and

Nutrition (book by Passwater, R. and Cranton, E.), 285
Truss, C. O., iii, v, vii, viii, 4, 13, 161, 167, 182, 198, 201, 207, 224, 225, 226, 251, 259, 265, 271, 275, 302

U

Ulene, Art, 92
Update (a quarterly periodical published by The Gesell Institute for Human Development), 259
Urethritis, 60, 233
  due to candida, 60
Urinary tract,
  problems of, 128, 174, 185, 236
  enuresis, 5
  frequency, 6, 60
  infections, 6, 14, 18, 184
    treatment of, 60, 200-201
  pain, 6, 60
Urticaria, 288-289 (see also hives)

V

Vaccines, yeast (see also Yeast-Connected Illness, treatment of, and Immunotherapy)
Vagina, 10
  anatomy of
    encourages yeast growth, 190
  cultures of,
    not helpful in diagnosis of yeast-connected health disorders, 27
  intravaginal therapy,
    Gyne-Lotrimin®, 44, 247
    Monistat-7®, 44, 247
    Mycelex G®, 247
    nystatin powder, 247
Vaginitis, vi, 12, 23, 28, 60, 178, 180, 181, 185, 187, 188, 232-235, 237,

239, 248, 294
  treatment with yogurt, 294
VanderWalt, Rika, 260
Vaporizers encourage mold growth, 57
Vegetables,
  as a source of carbohydrates, 43, 67, 70, 137
  contribution to a good diet for most people, vii, 67-72, 95, 137
  discussion of role in promoting yeast growth, 42, 43, 70, 71, 95
  fresh, 75, 93
Vegetable oils (see also Fatty acids, linseed oil, primrose oil)
  cold pressed, 85
  source of, 86
Vegetarianism, 69
Vibramycin®, 237 (see also Tetracyclines)
Viral infections, 12
Virgil, 291
Vision (see Eye problems)
Vitamin Diagnostics, Inc., 287
Vitamins,
  measures, 293
  supplements, 243, 244
Vitamin A,
  blood studies, 234
  deficiency of, 149, 234
  large doses of, 255
  safety of, 255
Vitamin B complex,
  supplements of, 138, 243, 290
Vitamin B-6,
  large doses helpful in treating premenstrual syndrome, 188, 288, 290
Vitamin C, 71, 194, 278
  as antioxidant or free radical scavenger, 285
  dosage of, 243, 244
    bowel tolerance test in determining, 244
  in asthma, 166, 244-245

in children with recurrent ear
infections, 210
in infections, 142
megadose of, 244-245, 278
powder, 244
strengthens the immune system,
165-166, 210, 245, 283
use by physicians, 278
use in relieving symptoms
caused by exposure to
chemicals & tobacco, 254-255
Vitamin E,
as antioxidant, 285
in premenstrual syndrome, 188,
290
Von Hilsheimer, George, 266
Vulvovaginitis, 60 (see also Vaginitis)

W

Waickman, Francis J., 4, 91, 199, 275
Wall Street Journal, 295
Ward, Walter, 272
Water, 90 ,150
bottled, 86
filters, 90-91
safety of, 90
Weakness, 22, 124
Web,
(illustration), 144, 219
the causes of illness resemble a,
145, 200, 219, 227, 254
Weight gain, excessive, 6, 71
Weight Watchers, 298
Western New York Allergy and
Ecology Association, 260
Wheezing, 174 (see also Asthma)
White Blood Cells, 9 (see also
Immune System)
Wholistic Medicine (see Holistic
Medicine)
Winger, Ed, 286-287
Williams, Roger J., 69, 165, 298
Willoughby, James, 265
Wollman, Leo, 291

Woman's Day (magazine), 298
Women, (see also Yeast-connected
illness and individual symptoms)
health problems of, 178-190
susceptibility to yeast-connected
illness, reasons for, 188-190
Women's National Health Network,
260
Worrell, Aubrey, 198
Worthen, Dennis B., 201

Y

Yeast, yeasts, 3, 10, 11, 19 (see also
molds)
definition of, 3
growth of encouraged by, (see also
diet, and yeast, dietary
management of)
antibiotics, 215
beer, 215
birth control pills, 215
fruits, 70-73, 215
grains, 119
hormonal changes, 215
milk, 215
sweets, 215
in diet,
comments on, 89-94, 118
in processed foods, 69, 85
overgrowth weakens immune
system, 11, 13, 15
sources, 42
tapes, 263
toxins, 11, 15, 197
types of, 3
Yeast-connected illness,
Birmingham Symposium on,
274-275
Dallas Conference on, 271-274
diagnosis of, 27, 28, 40
based on history, 27, 28, 272
use of questionnaires,
short, x
long, 29-33

dietary management of,
Candida Control Diet, 75-93
Fruit-free, Sugar-free, Yeast-free
Diet, 117-118
Fruit-free, Grain-free, Nut-free,
Milk-free Diet, 119-120
Low Carbohydrate Diet, 95-110
nutritional supplements,
essential fatty acids (see fatty
acids, essential)
minerals, (see minerals)
vitamins, (see Vitamins)
yeast-free diet, 41, 42, 43
How you Suspect, Identify and
Treat (Section A), 1-63
interest of the public in, 271
manifestations of, 177-240 (see also
separate listing of symptoms,
e.g., fatigue, headache,
depression, etc.)
in children, 42-43, 195-211
ear problems, 42, 59, 195, 196,
203-208
hyperactivity, 42, 195-198, 201,
202, 205-206
learning problems, 201, 195-198
in infants, 43
colic, 195, 202-203
ear problems, 42, 195
diaper rashes, persistent, 252
thrush, 252
in men, 40, 191-194, 291
in relationship to autism,
195-197, 289-290
in teenagers, 213-217
alcohol abuse, 213
anxiety, 214
crime, 213
depression, 213, 214
drug abuse, 213
erratic behavior, 213
headache, 214
short attention span, 214
suicide, 213
traffic accidents, 213

underachievement, 213
in women, 178-190, 191 (see
separate listing of symptoms
e.g. vaginitis, depression;
fatigue etc.)
predisposing factors, 15, 179
why more common, 188-190
mental disease, 289
muscle & joint, 25
nervous, 21, 22, 39, 43
respiratory, 25, 43
sex organ, 23, 39
skin, 23, 40
patience needed, in overcoming, 52
questions & answers, 39-52
questionnaire, 29-33
long, 29-33
short, x
recognition of,
role in controlling medical costs,
vi, 171-172
transmission of,
to spouse, 40, 252
treatment of, 35-37, 44-52
comprehensive program
important, 137-176, 273, 278,
279
effectiveness of, 278, 279
measures other than diet and
medication, 51, 131-175,
242-250, 277-300
attention and love, 143, 144,
145, 148 (see Psychological
factors)
allergy treatment, 141-142, 144,
145, 148
antioxidants, 285
avoid chemicals, 139-140, 144,
145, 148, 164
avoid junk food, 140-141, 144,
145, 165
avoid tobacco, 144
avoid toxins, 139-140, 144, 145,
148
candida extract, 224

essential fatty acids, 6, 141, 144,
148l
exercise, 143, 144, 148
favorable environment (light,
air, pure water), 142, 143,
144
garlic, 292
immunotherapy, 224
minerals, 138, 139, 144, 145,
148
molds, environmental, 165
psychological factors, 143, 144,
145, 148, 166
selenium, 285
strong immune system, 143,
148, 163-166
touch, 143, 148
treat bacterial infections, 142
vitamins, 138, 142, 144, 145,
148, 165
yogurt, 266, 267
medications,
amphotericin B, 50
clotrimazole, 50
ketoconazole (see Nizoral®)
Nizoral®, 48-50
nystatin, 44, 48 (see also
Nystatin)
vaccines, 51
observations of practicing
physicians, 277, 278
overcoming isn't always easy,
231-239
Yeast Connection, The . . . A Vicious
Cycle (chart), xvi
Yeast-free, Sugar-free, Fruit-free,
Nut-free, Milk-free diet, 73, 119
Yogurt, 251, 266
efficacy of in combatting
yeast-connected symptoms,
266-267
how to make, 267
Your Good Health (magazine), 299

Z

Zamm, Alfred, V., 4
Ziff, Michael F., 297
zinc, 138, 290, 291
in premenstrual syndrome, 188

Ordering Information

To order additional copies of *The Yeast Connection*, complete the following form and mail with check or money order to the address listed below:

FUTURE HEALTH, INC.
P. O. Box 846
Jackson, Tennessee 38302

For each copy ordered, please send $15.95 plus $2.05 per copy to cover postage and handling. Tennessee residents add .88 sales tax. Books cannot be mailed on credit; please send money order or check with this form.

SHIP TO:

Name: _____

Address: _____

_____

City: _____ State: _____ Zip: _____

Number of copies ordered: _____

Amount enclosed: $ _____

Method of payment: Check ☐   Money Order ☐